BEE PROPOLIS

BEE PROPOLIS

Natural Healing from the Hive

James Fearnley

SOUVENIR PRESS

This Edition published 2001 by
Souvenir Press Ltd.,
43 Great Russell Street, London WC1B 3PD

ISBN 0 285 63522 0

Typeset by Rowland Phototypesetting Ltd,
Bury St Edmunds, Suffolk

Printed in Great Britain by
The Guernsey Press Co. Ltd.,
Guernsey, Channel Islands

For my wife and family
Jackie and Rose, Lillah, Felix, Hugo, Cecily and Anna (Dorrie)

Contents

Acknowledgements

I can't believe how difficult it has been to write this little book about propolis—a product, which has consumed the last 9 years of my life. I could not have done it without the help and support of others.

I must thank all at the International Bee Research Association in Cardiff both for access to their superb database and for their personal and practical support. The encouragement and friendship of other propolis 'missionaries' in particular Bruce Brown and Linda Graham has been vital. Both their fathers did so much to put propolis on the map and both now continue 'the work' with equal zeal. Most of all I have to thank my wife Jackie and children Rose, Lillah, Felix, Hugo, Cecily and Dorrie for their endless patience and support.

Note to Readers

The aim of this book is to provide information on the uses of propolis in the treatment of relevant diseases. Although every care has been taken to ensure that the advice is accurate and practical, it is not intended to be a guide to self-diagnosis and self-treatment. Where health is concerned—and in particular a serious problem of any kind—it must be stressed that there is no substitute for seeking advice from a qualified medical or herbal practitioner. All persistent symptoms, of whatever nature, may have underlying causes that need, and should not be treated without, professional elucidation and evaluation.

It is therefore very important, if you are considering trying propolis for medicinal purposes, to consult your practitioner first, and if you are already taking any prescribed medication, do not stop it.

The Publisher makes no representation, express or implied, with regard to the accuracy of the information contained in this book, and legal responsibility or liability cannot be accepted by the Author or the Publisher for any errors or omissions that may be made or for any loss, damage, injury or problems suffered or in any way arising from following the advice offered in these pages.

INTRODUCTION

Propolis—Defender of the City

By way of the beehive the whole Cosmos enters man and makes him strong and able.

Rudolf Steiner,[1] *Nine Lectures on Bees*, 1923

The humble honeybee is a truly remarkable insect, producing a range of products upon which man has relied since time immemorial. Most of them we are familiar with—honey of course, royal jelly, pollen and bee venom. This book is about the renaissance of interest in one of the least-known products of the hive—propolis.

Propolis is a mainly resinous substance which bees collect from trees and plants. They take this resin back to the hive where other products, in particular wax, are added and the whole substance transformed into what we know as propolis. The word propolis, reputed to have been coined by Aristotle, takes its name from the Greek *pro* (before) *polis* (city)—'before the city' or 'defender of the city.'

Propolis has been used by man as a medicine since Egyptian times. But like the fairy tale princess Sleeping Beauty, propolis, in common with other natural medicines, has lain asleep for 'one hundred years', silent and forgotten. It has been surrounded by a forest of thorns—misunderstood, misrepresented, even derided, seen sometimes more as witchcraft than as the complex and powerful source of natural health that it is.

My own connection with propolis began nine years ago when I was introduced to it by a beekeeper in Whitby, North Yorkshire. At the time, I was running a wholefood shop selling a variety of natural health products. When I began to explore the history and use of propolis I quickly realised that here was a substance with an apparently astonishing range of therapeutic qualities. The more I studied the available literature the more I realised that if only half what was said about it was true then here was a product which more people should know about and have available to them.

The seven years since that meeting have been a fascinating voyage of discovery about this complex substance. They have also been a rollercoaster of commercial activity during which time propolis has emerged from the dusty back shelves of health food shops to become a major-selling, high-profile health product worth several million pounds in the UK market alone. The 'hobby' business which started as a result of a chance meeting has become an all-consuming passion which has taken me to almost every continent on earth in search of raw materials, research or markets for a business which has 'growed' like Topsy.

The renewal of interest in propolis has come at a time when natural medicine is growing exponentially, partly because of an awakening interest in all manner of natural ways of staying well and combating disease, but also as a result of an increasing concern with the side effects of chemical medicine. In particular, the over-prescribing of antibiotics is now perceived by the public as a significant problem with modern drug-based medicine.

The public as a whole is now aware that antibiotics are not the 'magic bullet' answer we first thought them to be. Serious problems of bacterial resistance are being revealed. Bacteria have shown they have a remarkable talent to mutate and adapt to the stronger and ever more sophisticated drugs developed to combat them. Immune deficiency diseases have become one of the dominant concerns of modern medicines throughout the world. The search is on for effective solutions to a wide range of both new diseases and, more alarmingly, old ones re-emerging.

Dr George Jacoby,[2] of Harvard Medical School, puts the problem succinctly: 'Bugs are always figuring out ways to get around the antibiotics we throw at them . . . They adapt, then come roaring back.' Dr Harold Neu[3], of Columbia University, is even more direct: 'Bacteria are cleverer than man.' Laurie Garret,[4] in her outstanding analysis of changing patterns of disease worldwide, *The Coming Plague*, claims that man has been 'lulled into complacency born of proud discoveries and medical triumph, unprepared for the coming plague'.

The real scale of the health crisis we face is impossible to quantify but it is certain that the problem relates not just to antibiotic drugs but also to a whole range of orthodox allopathic drugs including anti-fungal, anti-inflammatory and antiviral drugs.

Propolis has been shown to have antibiotic, anti-inflammatory, anti-fungal antioxidant and antiviral properties all rolled into one, with virtually no known side effects. It is not difficult to understand why, when claims like this are made for natural products, they are often met with derision by orthodox medicine. To suggest that a natural product may have a single function, as an antibiotic perhaps, or as an anti-inflammatory, may seem plausible, but to suggest that this sticky, resinous glue, produced by bees to bung up holes in the hive, can help with everything from AIDS to asthma is like suggesting that your pet donkey can win the Grand National.

However, the purpose of this book is not to seek converts for natural medicine as against orthodox allopathic medicine. It is simply to inform as many people as possible about a product they may know little of, in order that they can decide for themselves what they think of it and whether it can be of use to them.

CHAPTER 1

What is Propolis?

Propolis is composed principally of resin and wax. Its colour can vary enormously. In temperate climates it ranges from a light yellow or brown to a dark brown colour, often with a reddish hue. Propolis produced in tropical climates can range from the light brown-green of Brazilian propolis to the black and dark red of some Cuban varieties. Propolis tends to become darker the longer it is in the hive. Fresh propolis appears as a red tinge on the new white comb constructed by the bees. The colour of propolis also varies according to the trees and plants harvested, as well as the types of bees gathering it. Propolis collected by black bees tends to be darker in colour.

You can find propolis most easily at two sites in the hive—at the entrance, which is constructed almost entirely from propolis, and along the sides of the frames, where it is often deposited in larger quantities in zigzag patterns. Some believe these larger deposits act as a kind of storage facility before being moved to fill cracks or openings, or to be rendered down into a finer, more liquid form for use elsewhere in the hive.

At moderate temperatures propolis becomes soft and malleable when handled but when frozen becomes brittle. Propolis turns to a liquid at temperatures between 70–100°C.

HOW DO BEES COLLECT PROPOLIS?

Most beekeepers and researchers now believe that the resins in propolis are collected directly by the bees from trees, shrubs and plants. However, this is not the only theory that has been put forward. In 1907 Kustenmacher,[1] a German bee researcher, suggested that propolis was largely derived from pollen granules.

Kustenmacher believed that that the bees took pollen granules into a section of their intestine where the granules would swell to five times their size as they absorbed water. As the granules burst open they released a plasma which he believed the bees used to feed their young.

The pollen husks that remained were processed into a balsam, which was then excreted. This balsamic excretion was then mixed with other discarded pollen husks, waxes and detritus from the hive, forming the basis of propolis. The resulting more solid, brownish mixture could then be transported around the hive. Support for this theory has come from some experiments, which show that even where bees are deprived of resinous materials but not pollen, propolis is still produced. Further support also comes from the observation that maximum production of propolis always coincides with times of greatest pollen production.

Whilst not all of Kustenmacher's theory has been discarded, the advent of modern biochemical analysis has very much weakened it. For example, research has shown that few, if any, of the chemicals released in the breakdown of pollen end up in propolis.

By far the most plausible and now most popular theory was put forward by Rosch[2] and others, again in the early part of this century. Rosch observed bees removing sections of resin from trees with their mandibles, which they used to further break down the resinous lumps. The resin was then passed from the forelegs to the mid-legs of the bee, continuing to be worked on and gradually formed into a pellet as pollen is, before being deposited into the bee's pollen baskets. The bees then flew back to the hive where other bees removed the propolis and transferred it to storage sites or applied it in the hive for a variety of purposes.

A combination of the two theories was suggested by Phillip[3] in the 1930s. He argued that there were two kinds of propolis, one produced in the way described by Kustenmacher and the second, according to Rosch, by the collection of resin from external sources. Phillip maintained that the propolis produced from pollen had the most important use in the hive, covering and sterilizing the cells into which the queen lays her eggs. Propolis collected from external sources had a secondary use, more as a building material within the hive—strengthening the comb and filling cracks and crevices. Personally, I feel that there may be something in the Phillip theory which does explain the two different uses of propolis, but I think we will have to wait for further, one imagines difficult, research, for a definitive answer.

THE IMPORTANCE OF RESINS

One thing is certain—resins derived from one source or another, form a major ingredient, around 50 per cent, of propolis. From the outset, the bees are collecting a material which the plant world already relies on to maintain its health and integrity.

We know resins have an important role to play in the immune defence systems of trees and plants. We have all seen how, if a tree is damaged or cut, the resins pour out in order to seal up the 'wound', to stop the tree bleeding. Many of these resins themselves have a hallowed place in natural medicines. Two out of the three gifts taken by the Wise Men to the infant Jesus at his birth were tree resins—frankincense and myrrh. Frankincense and myrrh have well-documented anti-inflammatory properties and are used to treat a variety of health problems, including rheumatism and arthritis, as well as for bronchial and respiratory complaints. Other resins, including poplar bud resin, benzoin and pine resin, have figured in their own right as part of the natural medicine chest, for similar reasons. It is not surprising therefore that the honeybee should seek out these and other resins as a valuable base material for propolis.

DO BEES CREATE SOMETHING UNIQUE IN PROPOLIS?

How much the bees work on the resins they collect from trees and plants, transforming them into propolis by processing them both outside and inside the hive, is still a matter of debate. Some researchers believe the bees take an active part in transforming resin into propolis with the help of glandular secretions produced as they collect the resin.[4] These secretions contain enzymes which metabolise the resin. A Cuban study in 1990[5] showed that the resins collected by the bees are at least in part metabolised by them, and Greenaway[6] in 1997 suggests that by adding saliva during the scraping and chewing of the resins, new elements, e.g. sugars, are produced. The same research showed that the chemical structure of the bioflavonoids in tree resins collected by the bees is changed by the time they appear in propolis. Others researchers argue that it is the tree or plant resins, pure and simple, which give propolis its unique protective and therapeutic properties within the beehive. My own feeling is that the extraordinary capacity of the honeybee to transform a range of simple raw materials, pollen and nectar for example, into highly complex substances like honey and royal jelly supports the idea that the bee is actively contributing to the creation of something new and unique.

The beehive is a symbol of how simpler substances derived from the lower order of the plant world are elevated and transformed by the bee into substances appropriate for a higher order of existence. In comparing the wide range of therapeutic properties which propolis provides for man with the often narrower range of therapeutic properties possessed by single plants or herbs, we are made aware again of the quantum leap in complexity and sophistication which differentiates the plant from the animal world.

THE POPLAR TREE MYTH

One commonly held belief about the origin of propolis is that it is derived solely from the resin of the poplar tree. This is not the case. Although the poplar tree is a favoured source of resin, where available, bees will collect from a wide variety of trees, shrubs and plants depending on what is locally available. Why bees choose one source above another remains a mystery. We can only assume that bees possess a sense of attraction which guides them to those trees, shrubs or plants most able to provide them with the structural and pharmacological properties they need.

NOT ALL BEES COLLECT PROPOLIS

Only the Western honeybee (*Apis mellifera*) is known to forage for propolis whilst the Asian species of honeybee do not. *Apis mellifera* is present throughout the world and it is clear that it is able to adapt to whatever flora is available to collect the resins essential for propolis. The colour, smell and composition of propolis is determined by the dominant sources of resins in the region.

Some tropical bees, *Apis cerana, Apis dorsata* and Tropical *Apis mellifera*, make no use of propolis at all, and Carniolan bees are reported to use wax instead of propolis. The tropical stingless bees or *Meliponine* do collect a resinous substance similar to propolis, which they use to seal up the hive and to create honey and pollen storage vessels. However, little is known about this species and by far the bulk of research into propolis has been conducted into *Apis mellifera.*

Exactly why some bees collect propolis and others do not remains unclear. Is it perhaps because some bees do not require the sterilising, antibiotic properties that propolis provides or do they utilise other products for these purposes? Could it be that Phillips and Kustenmacher are right after all and that the most important sterilising function in the hive is provided by propolis derived from the breakdown of pollen? May it also be that bees which are truly native to southern climates do not have the same need for, and therefore have not evolved a system for collecting, the cruder 'double glazing' variety of externally-gathered propolis. Perhaps where they have a need for a building material rather than an antibiotic material, instead of using resin they substitute other materials like soil and other debris, as do the stingless bees of Africa or use wax alone as do Carniolan bees.

Cuban researchers are currently looking at the reasons why propolis produced in the southern hemisphere by the Western *Apis mellifera* contains a different package of microelements to that produced in the northern hemisphere. It may be that this work will somehow lead us to a better understanding of why other types of bees, which are truly indigenous to tropical climates, do not produce propolis at all.

We must assume evolution plays some part in the propolis story. Some bees, we know, are noted for collecting propolis more actively than others; in particular Grey Mountain Caucasian bees collect more than dark forest bees. Italian, Ukranian and Far East bees collect very little propolis Theo Frederich,[7] a beekeeper on Vancouver Island, British Columbia, tells us that, 'today's bees propolize less than they used to, many of us will remember the old days with the old black bees that glued everything solid, when you could literally scrape off a quarter pound of propolis from the entrances.' He goes on to tell us that those modern beekeepers have bred queens specifically to produce less propolis in order to make their job easier.

WHAT DOES PROPOLIS CONTAIN?

Whether or not there are two distinct forms of propolis the majority of research which has explored its components, has been carried on propolis harvested externally. Whilst resin and wax are the two major ingredients, research, particularly over the last 15 years has revealed an increasingly complex package of additional microelements. In 1990, at Oxford, Greenaway[8] identified 150 distinct compounds in propolis. More recent studies have identified a further 30 new compounds. As our chemical analytical equipment improves, so further biochemical dimensions of propolis are revealed and it seems likely that more elements yet remain to be discovered.

The constituents of propolis can vary considerably according to where in the world the propolis is harvested and the plants and trees the bees have visited. Content can also vary according to season of collection and even the time of the day the bees collect the resins. Table 1 shows the five major compounds in propolis

Table 1: The Principal Compounds in Propolis

Resins	45–55%
Waxes and fatty acids	25–35%
Essential oils	10%
Pollen	5%
Other organics and minerals	5%

The resins contain the majority of the flavonoids—perhaps as many as 40—found in propolis along with a number of phenols and acids. Flavonoids are found everywhere in the plant kingdom, especially in fruit and vegetables. Propolis contains particularly high quantities of a large range of flavonoids and it is these that have attracted most attention from researchers seeking the so-called 'actives' in propolis, i.e. those elements thought most responsible for particular pharmacological actions. We shall return for a more detailed look at the role of flavonoids later when we look at the pharmacological and physiological effects of propolis.

Most of the waxes and fatty acids present in propolis are derived from beeswax but many of them are of plant origin. The role of the waxes in propolis has been neglected. When propolis is refined the waxes are generally removed. They are, however, an integral and important part of propolis and contain a range of micro-elements thought to be important in treating burns. Clinical trials using beeswax to treat burns are currently being carried out in a hospital in the south of England.

The range of essential oils found in propolis depends on the flora harvested by the bees. Petri,[9] a Hungarian researcher, has compared the essential oils collected from propolis with the oil from poplar bud, that favourite source of resin for the bees. Microbiological tests showed similar moderate activity against some bacteria and fungi.

The small amount of pollen found in propolis is responsible for its protein content. Gabrys,[10] a Polish researcher, found 16 amino acids present in propolis at more than 1 per cent. Of the total amino acids present, arginine and proline together made up 45.8 per cent. A further eight amino acids were present in traces. Gabrys suggests that the ability of propolis to stimulate tissue regeneration is due to the presence of arginine because of its role in stimulating the production of nucleic acid.

Around 14 mineral trace elements are found in propolis, of which iron and zinc are the most common. Other minerals found include gold, silver, caesium, mercury and lead.

In 1994 high levels of lead were found in propolis on sale to consumers in the UK. Explanations for this ranged from atmospheric pollution to the use of hives painted with lead paint. Paradoxically however, it appears that resin has an unusual affinity for lead and may even remove it from the body. Felix Murat[11] in his book *Propolis—The Eternal Natural Healer*, tells an interesting story of how lead ingested from car exhaust fumes in Athens can be eliminated from the body by drinking the local wine, retsina! Murat explains that when the grapes are pressed and the wine first starts to ferment, 'a certain amount of virgin resin, fresh as it comes from the tapped pine trees, is poured into the fermenting vat.' The resin in retsina, with its affinity for lead, and also mercury, absorbs the metal, turning it into harmless compounds which are eliminated through urination.

By a strange twist the most advanced propolis refining plant in the world, recently built in Arizona and developed to remove lead and other heavy metals from propolis, utilises newly developed supercolloidal technology which involves passing liquid propolis through a column charged with resin. The lead particles are selectively attracted to the resin. Perhaps the real question here, however, is whether the metals, like lead, which propolis appears to attract are there for some positive purpose or whether this natural affinity just happens to be operating as a natural collector of lead in the environment.

Finally, a variety of additional organic compounds are also found in propolis. These include ketones, lactones, quinones, steroids, benzoic acid and esters, vitamins and sugars. As research adds further elements to the growing list of those already known to be in propolis, so the biochemical and pharmacological mystery of propolis deepens. But before we explore this mystery as it relates to our health, let's remain a little longer with the bee itself and examine how it uses propolis in the hive.

CHAPTER 2

The Role of Propolis in the Hive

In between acting as teacher to Alexander the Great and writing his great works on ethics and philosophy, Aristotle (384–322 BC) found time to write the first detailed natural scientific study of animals. This work included substantial and detailed references to the working of the honeybee. Aristotle's great goal was to understand the intimate workings of the hive and in particular the role of the 'mother bee' or, as we know it, the queen bee.[1]

Aristotle recognised two types of propolis and had clearly arrived at a detailed understanding of their role and purpose. *Conosis* propolis, he tells us, is used by the bees to fill cracks and holes in the hive, keeping out the light, weather and potential intruders such as spiders, ants and other insects which might wish to invade the warmth, shelter and food supply of the hive. *Mitys* propolis, on the other hand, was a richer, darker, more aromatic substance. This was used to narrow the entrance to the hive and was also used in the cell walls.

Ad Amiri,[2] an Arab writing some years later, provides us with a revealing insight both into the way Aristotle worked as a scientist and into the use made of propolis. In his attempt to observe the bees at work, Aristotle built an observation hive made of glass. But the bees did not approve and refused to work until they had smeared the inside of the glass with a dark, sticky substance, a clear reference to the use of propolis to block out the light in the hive.

THE BEES' EXTERNAL IMMUNE SYSTEM?

The role of propolis in the hive is linked to a central conundrum. How does a colony of bees, usually of 50,000 or more, crowded into a virtually hermetically-sealed space, at a constant temperature of 35°C (95°F) and with moisture levels of 90 per cent, manage to survive? Surely these conditions are perfect for the growing of bacteria and the spreading of disease, and yet bees have not only survived but prospered in such conditions for millions of years. In many ways, conditions in the hive mirror conditions in the human body (the brood-rearing temperature is actually the same as our body temperature) and present similar problems—constant high temperature and levels of moisture. The answer for us humans is that we have our complex immune defence mechanism, while the bees use propolis.

Dramatic as this may sound it is hard to avoid the conclusion that propolis effectively provides a form of externalised immune defence mechanism for the beehive, fulfilling its role in a multitude of ways. It does this at times by using very simple, practical, structural mechanisms. At other times it involves highly complex, pharmacological processes, aspects of which are as yet not entirely understood.

DEFENDING THE CITY

The labyrinthine passageway into the hive, the entrance to the city, incorporates both mechanisms. The winding passageway is built entirely of propolis. It should provide the only entrance into the hive. Through it must pass all the bee traffic between the hive and the outside world. Practically and structurally, by narrowing the entrance down with propolis the entrance can be defended by the—guard bees against intruders—mainly other bees, ants and other insects. But it defends the hive in another more subtle way. Being made out of resin, it also acts as a kind of sterilizing chamber through which all the bees must pass—a long, narrow and circuitous chamber which slowly cleanses the bees of bacteria as they move towards the heart of the hive and an environment which is recognised as the most sterile known in nature.

As we have seen from Aristotle's observations the honeybee does not like to be exposed to the light. In the wild, bees will build their hives in protected spaces like hollow tree trunks, caves or crevices. In urban environments they may seek the safety of roof spaces, as they have done in my own home in North Yorkshire, or redundant chimneys as one colony did many years ago at the offices of the International Bee Research Association in Cardiff! Propolis is used to seal up the unprotected sides of the colony, keeping out the light as well as providing protection from the weather and intruders.

In commercial hives bees seek to protect themselves in a similar way, sealing up any external holes in the hive and closing any internal gaps which may cause unhealthy draughts, for example between the frames and the hive walls. However, they also use propolis to create the right amount of air circulation in the hive by restricting or enlarging, according to need, 'ventilation' holes through which air can enter from outside.

Beekeepers groan when you mention propolis. For most of them it is not a valuable natural medicine but rather a huge nuisance which increases their work in managing the bees and collecting the honey, by firmly gluing all the moveable parts of the hive to each other and to the hive walls. We have already heard how some beekeepers have tried to breed this tendency out of the bees. With current demand for good-quality propolis running high perhaps they should be doing the reverse.

Inevitably, however, not all would-be intruders into the hive are deterred by the natural fortification provided by propolis. Felix Murat[3] tells us of one variety of bees, *Apis florea*, which has a particular problem with ants. These ants have worked out that they stand no chance singly against the bees guarding the hive entrance so they have evolved a counter-strategy. They gather *en masse* near to the hive and then swoop on the hive entrance. Some ants are stung to death by the guards but inevitably the sheer numbers of ants are able to overwhelm them. When this happens the ants enter the hive killing the queen and removing everything edible, including larvae, honey and other bees. *Apis florea* however, not to be outdone, has itself devised a countermeasure. The bees smear propolis all over the area surrounding the entrance to the hive, creating something resembling a giant fly trap, or in this case ant trap. The invading ants stick fast in the propolis and can be more easily stung and killed. The dead ants are then coated with propolis and can remain effectively mummified, sometimes in heaps around the entrance to the hive, until they are consumed by the voracious larvae of the wax moth which lays its eggs in beehives.

DEALING WITH INVADERS

Unfortunately, not all intruders are kept out of the hive. Bees and other insects as well as snails and small animals—frogs, mice and lizards—sometimes find their way into the hive in search of warmth and food. In the case of smaller insects this is not too much of a problem. They can be stung to death and even physically removed. It is the demise of the larger intruders which provides the most graphic and symbolic illustration of how propolis protects the body of the hive from infection. In the case of a mouse, for example, the bees may be able to sting it to death but cannot hope to remove it. Left to rot, the dead mouse would present a serious bacterial problem within the hive. The colony responds to the threat with a rapid transfer of all available propolis to the site of the corpse where they proceed to cover every exposed surface of the dead mouse, finally giving it a top coating of wax. The mouse, like the ants caught outside the hive, is effectively mummified, sealed up within the hive. The process of decomposition is stopped, the corpse is no longer a threat to the colony.

The role of propolis at this macro level is mirrored on a micro level within the hive. When we come to look at the pharmacological properties of propolis we will see how bacteria in the hive are not simply destroyed or annihilated as they might be by synthetic antibiotics; rather, they are surrounded, neutralised and disarmed in the same way as the mouse is—a powerful metaphor of the relationship between the natural and the man-made.

A HIGH-TECH BUILDING MATERIAL

Perhaps the least-known but most intriguing aspect of the role of propolis in the hive is its use as a building material. In 1964 a Russian scientist, J. K. Leipus,[4] worked out that 1 lb of beeswax honeycomb was capable of holding 25 lbs of honey which, in engineering terms, makes honeycomb a remarkable substance. The interlocking hexagonal cells no doubt contribute something to the honeycomb's strength but he suggests it is propolis which enables the comb to carry the load it does. 90–95 per cent of the comb is made of beeswax while the remainder is composed of propolis. The propolis acts like a natural 'carbon fibre' reinforcement both within the cell itself and in connecting it with surrounding cells. Leipus also demonstrated that all the brood cells and honey cells were coated with a very thin but complete layer of propolis resin. Apart from the sterilizing function of this lining the naturally impervious and adhesive tension of the resinous envelope probably also adds to the internal strengthening of each cell. It is interesting that resins are being incorporated in a new generation of building materials for the construction industry and that they are noted for their high-tensile and load-bearing properties. It seems once again that nature got there first.

STERILIZING THE HIVE

Inside the hive, propolis is used in its most complex pharmaceutical form. A very fine resinous material is used to 'polish' and effectively sterilize every surface in the hive. It is particularly important that the brood cells into which the queen will lay her eggs are bacteria-free. The queen bee can lay upwards of 3,000 eggs per day—over twice her own body weight. The worker bees ensure that every cell into which an egg is placed is lined with propolis. Ghisalberti,[5] in his 1979 review of propolis, has suggested that an additional reason for coating the cells with propolis is to provide an impervious lining, limiting the escape of water vapour needed for the developing brood. Once the eggs have been laid, a wax and propolis mixture is used to cap each cell, providing a final antibiotic and anti-fungal seal. Even the honeybee's most determined bacterial enemy, *Bacillus larvae*—the cause of American Foul Brood,[6,7] has been shown to succumb to propolis. The cells into which honey is stored receive a similar treatment—lined first with propolis and then capped with wax and propolis. A traditional and highly effective remedy for bronchitis was for the sufferer to eat the comb cappings after the honey had been extracted.

One cannot help but marvel at the ingenuity and wisdom of the honeybee in the way it utilises propolis in so comprehensive and effective way within the hive.

CHAPTER 3

The Folk History and Use of Propolis

Propolis has been used by man for a variety of medicinal and non-medicinal purposes since ancient times. It is tempting to think that before modern science the ancients were somehow forced to use natural substances as a kind of last resort, because they knew no better. The truth was very different and as we review the history of propolis we need to examine again our whole mindset relating to how our ancestors understood and worked with nature.

Whilst the ancients may not have had the technology and language of modern science, they certainly had knowledge. But it was a different, no less powerful knowledge, derived from a different worldview and sense of being. Their worldview was based on a relationship with and understanding of nature, gained through perception and intuition as well as through pure observation. It was a worldview which experienced and understood natural phenomenon as part of a powerful, unified and ultimately divine system.

THE EGYPTIANS

In ancient Egypt the priests were also the scientists, keeping sacred their knowledge of the natural world and its chemistry, and using this knowledge in medicine, engineering or agriculture. The land of Canaan, the Bible tells us, was a land 'flowing with milk and honey' and was one of the earliest areas where agriculture and cattle rearing were practised. There would be plenty of food for the honeybee. The Egyptians' capacity for detailed observation of nature is illustrated by the many anatomically accurate sketches of the honeybee that can be found in wall paintings still extant.

Around 3500 BC when Upper and Lower Egypt were united under one ruler, the bee was used as a symbol to denote the ruler of Upper Egypt, whilst the reed denoted the ruler of Lower Egypt. The Kahun papyrus[1] refers to this political union.

> He hath united the two lands,
> He hath joined the Reed to the Bee.

Pliny, the Roman writer, noted that the resin in propolis could be collected from, amongst other sources, the reed, making the symbolism of the Egyptian unification even more potent.

The Egyptians believed that the dead would need their bodies in the next life. Mummification was designed to preserve the body after death, intact as far as possible, for this event. To do this the priests used bee products extensively. First, the body was prepared by the removal of certain of the internal organs. Then the priests would soak the body itself, and the bandages with which they wrapped it, in a mixture produced by melting down the whole honeycomb—a combination of wax, honey and propolis. In surviving records it is clear that while the Egyptians distinguished between honey and wax they had no special term for the propolis itself, unlike the Greeks.

Modern research has confirmed the antibiotic and preservative qualities of honey and more especially of propolis. This may explain why the mummies, like the mummified mice that are found in hives, have been preserved intact for thousands of years. Numerous descriptions exist of how the Egyptians preserved their dead in honey, sealing the coffins with wax. One story provides a particularly graphic illustration of this practice. Robbers seeking treasure in one of the pyramids found a sealed jar containing honey. One of the robbers dipping his bread into the honey found a human hair. On closer inspection they found the body of a small child still intact, complete with ornaments, and perfectly preserved in its honey-filled tomb.[2]

Mysterious healing properties were attributed to these mummified remains. Those touching them were said to be cured of many diseases. So powerful was the belief, that in the absence of the real thing, mummies were created specifically for the purposes. An ancient Persian manuscript describes how you can make one yourself.[3]

> Find a ruddy, red-haired man and feed him till he is three years old on fruit; then drown him in a stone vessel which is filled with honey and drugs and seal up the vessel. When it is opened after the lapse of one hundred and fifty years, the honey will have turned the body into a mummy.

The interesting reference to the inclusion of 'drugs' may well refer to a folk knowledge of propolis as a healing agent already tried and tested by the priests in Egypt.

The Sumerians, and later the Babylonians, also used honey to preserve their dead. 'They bury their dead in honey and have funeral lamentations like the Egyptians,' said one writer.[4] Another chronicler recorded that, 'The Assyrians bury the body in honey first smearing it with wax.'

In a modern biography of Alexander the Great the author tells us how on his deathbed Alexander ordered that he be buried in honey.[5] This was done using 'white honey, which had not been melted.' With Aristotle as his teacher, Alexander would no doubt have been aware of the preserving properties of honey and propolis.

The Syriac Book of Medicine contains interesting references to what today we would understand as the powerful anti-bacterial role of propolis in the hive. These references were presented as a series of handy tips to Syrian beekeepers for maintaining a healthy beehive and therefore a good honey supply. Two of the tips in particular remind us yet again of our mouse story. Syrian beekeepers were advised to 'bury the liver of a white falcon in a beehive and the bees will thrive'. It was also suggested that 'whosoever shall place the eye of a bear in a hive of working bees, the bees shall prosper.'[6]

The presence of dead, potentially decomposing matter within the hive would present a serious bacterial problem. The bees would respond by producing fresh propolis as well as calling on existing stores to seal up the foreign matter. By stimulating the production of propolis we can see how the bees' 'immune response' mechanism was triggered, leading to improved all-round health in the hive. One is reminded here of the current use of bee venom injected directly into the bloodstream to boost the immune system of sufferers of post-viral fatigue syndrome.

THE GREEKS

It was not until Greek times that we find the first specific reference to propolis, in Aristotle's pioneering natural scientific study of the honeybee, and it was the Greeks who first took up beekeeping as an agricultural activity. By around 400 BC, during the time of Pericles, 20,000 beehives were kept in Attica, an area which became famous for its honey, believed to possess medicinal properties.[7]

The Greeks continued to use honey to embalm and preserve human bodies, particularly those of their soldiers who died far from home. Agesipolis, the Spartan king, who died in Asia, was preserved in honey like Alexander the Great before him, before being brought home to Sparta. Not only soldiers could demand this treatment; the Greek philosopher Democritus was also preserved in honey following his death.

Hippocrates (460–377 BC), considered by many the father of modern medicine, recognised the medicinal properties of propolis and is reputed to have prescribed propolis to help heal sores and ulcers, both external and internal.

The Greeks used propolis as the principal ingredient of a reputedly exquisite perfume called 'polyanthus'. The recipe combined finely mixed propolis with olibanum styrax, benzoin and aromatic herbs. It was burnt on slow-burning charcoal and apparently produced a wonderfully delicate and aromatic incense.[8]

THE ROMANS

The Romans were responsible for the further development of beekeeping and for extending our understanding of propolis. The exact origin of propolis was the subject of dispute between Pliny,[7] the prolific researcher and writer on natural history, and the doctor, Dioscorides. Pliny thought that propolis was resin harvested by the bees from the buds of willow, elm and reed and other plants, whilst Dioscorides thought it was harvested solely from *Styrax*.

Pliny in his 35-volume *Natural History* illustrated a considerable knowledge of the bee world including a detailed understanding of propolis.

> First they construct combs and mould wax, that is, construct their homes and cells, then produce offspring, and afterwards honey, wax from flowers, bee-glue from the droppings of the gum-producing trees—the sap, glue and resin of the willow, elm and reed. They first smear the whole interior of the hive itself with these as with a kind of stucco, and then with other bitterer juices as a protection against the greed of other small creatures, as they know that they are going to make something that may possibly be coveted; with the same materials they also build wider gateways round the structure.

Pliny goes on to define three separate types of propolis. The first is *Commosis* from which the word 'cosmetic' is derived. This is a thin varnish-like substance, which the bees use to paint, polish and disinfect all the surfaces in the hive. Then comes *Pissoceros*, a mixture of propolis resin and wax, which the bees use as a building material to seal holes and to reinforce the comb. Finally, he identifies *Propolis* itself, so-called because the bees use it to construct the narrow winding entrance to the hive—the true Defender of the City.

Pliny also refers to the medicinal properties of propolis:

> current physicians use propolis as a medicine because it extracts stings and all substances embedded in the flesh, reduces swelling, softens indurations (hardened tissue), soothes pains of the sinews and heals sores when it appears hopeless of them to mend.

Dioscorides, a leading Roman authority on healing, writing in the first century AD, refers frequently in his *Materia Medica* to the use of honey, wax and propolis in treating illness.

> The yellow bee glue that is of a sweet scent and resembling styrax, is to be chosen, and which is soft in ye excessive

> dryness of it, and easy to spread after the fashion of mastic. It is extremely warm and attractive, and (is good for the) drawing out of thorns and splinters. And being suffumigated it doth help old coughs and being applied it doth take away the lichens. It is found about ye mouths of hives, in nature like unto wax.[10]

Celsus, writing in the same period, includes propolis in a list of products able to 'mature abcessions and promote suppuration:' they were:

> nard, myrrh, costmary, balsal, galbanum propolis, styrax, frankincense, both the root and the bark, bitumen, pitch sulphur, resin, suet, fat, oil. . . . The best extractive, however, is that called by the Greeks rhypodes, from its resemblance to dirt. It contains myrrh, crocus, iris, propolis, bedelium, pomegranate heads, alum, mistletoe juice, turpentine resin or he-goat's suet.[11]

THE ARAB WORLD

References to the religious significance of the bee abound in ancient civilizations, often in relation to health and healing. Even with the coming of Islam and its disapproval of pantheistic cults we find references to the power of the honeybee and the medicinal properties of the hive.

> Thy Lord has taught the bee saying 'provide thee houses in the mountains and in the trees, and in the hives which men do build for thee. Feed, moreover, on every kind of fruit, and walk the beaten paths of the Lord.' From its belly comes forth a fluid of varying hues, which yieldeth medicine for men.[12]

Ibn Magih, an Arabic writer, quotes Mohammed as saying: 'Honey is a remedy for every illness, and the Koran is a remedy for all illness of the mind, therefore I recommend to you both remedies, the Koran and Honey.'

The Arab doctor Abu Ali ibn Sina (Avicenna)[13] in his famous book The Canon of Medicine spoke of two different kinds of wax—clean wax and black wax. It seems clear that the black wax was propolis which, according to Avicenna, 'has the characteristics of eliminating the spikes of the bolts and the stakes. It also rarefies, cleans and soaks.' As an aside he also tells us that 'by its strong smell, the black wax makes you sneeze.'

PROPOLIS IN EUROPE

Very few direct references to propolis are found in early British herbal literature. There are, however, numerous references to the anti-inflammatory properties of tree and plant resins, the basic raw materials harvested by the bee to produce propolis.

John Gerard[14] in his famous Herball refers to 'the rosin or clammie substance of the blacke Poplar buds.' He tells us how the apothecaries used these substances to make ointments for treating a range of inflammatory conditions.

Nicholas Culpeper,[15] in his *Complete Herbal*, also refers to the medicinal properties of poplar tree resin. 'The clammy buds hereof, before they spread into leaves, are gathered to make Unguentum and Populneum . . . The ointment called Populneum, which is made of this Poplar, is singularly good for all heat and inflammation in any part of the body and tempers the heat of wounds.'

In Green's *Universal Herbal*[16] we find further references to the use of the resin from two species of poplar trees. Under *Populus nigra* (Black Poplar Tree) Green tells us:

> The young leaves are an excellent ingredient for poultices for hard and painful swellings. The buds of both this and the White Poplar smell very pleasantly and being pressed between the fingers, yield balsamic resinous substances which, extracted by spirits of wine, smells like styrax. A drachm of this tincture in broth is administered in internal ulcers and excoriations and is said to have removed obstinate fluxes proceeding from an excoriation of the intestine.

Under *Populus balsamifera* (Common Tacamahaca Poplar Tree) we hear:

> 'The buds of this tree from autumn to the leafing are covered with an abundance of glutinous yellow balsam, which often collects into drops, and is pressed from the tree as a medicine. It dissolves in the spirits of wine; and the inhabitants of Siberia prepare a medicated wine from the buds. This wine is diuretic and, as they think serviceable in the scurvy.'[17]

Whilst very little appears to have been known about propolis in Britain and northern Europe it seems that in old southern and central Russia propolis was a familiar natural remedy. It is interesting to speculate whether this knowledge had always existed in these areas or whether it traveled north from Greece and the Arab countries.

In Georgia, where the Arab influence was strong, Sul-han-Saba (1658–1725) the complier of a Georgian encyclopedic dictionary defined propolis as 'a substance similar to wax from the bottom of the hive.'[18]

In the *Carabadini*,[19] a Georgian book of medicine published in the thirteenth century, the author suggests a treatment for dental decay. The recipe involves propolis mixed with arsenic, red lentil, yarrow, wood germander, to which is added one spoon of olive oil and one of honey. The mixture is then placed on the bad tooth. Propolis as we shall see later is now used extensively by modern dentists to treat a wide variety of periodontal problems.

Moving towards modern times another Georgian medical treatise, published in the 18th century, recommends the use of propolis for the treatment of haemoptysis. 'One has to take propolis grains having the size of a pin's head, for two days—three pieces, in the morning and in the afternoon.'[20]

Traditionally, in Georgia, propolis cakes—small flat pats of propolis—were used to treat a variety of conditions. For arthritis the cake was wrapped in a warm cloth and left on the inflamed or painful area all night. A similar treatment was recommended for treating skin abscesses, where it is claimed the propolis cake eliminated the pus very quickly.[21] For treating corns a thin layer of propolis was placed on the corn and then bandaged into place. Parents of newborn children were also advised to place a propolis cake on the belly button of newborn children and to rub their children's toys with propolis.

A. B. Nikolaev[22] refers to a traditional Georgian treatment for respiratory tract infections where finely ground propolis is inhaled by the sufferer.

CHAPTER 4

Propolis in Modern Times

For thousands of years natural medicine—herbs and plants to treat disease—was the only medicine available to humans. As we have seen, medicine then was as much allied to a religious worldview as modern drug-based medicine is to scientific thinking. However, from the middle of the eighteenth century onwards little of the old medicine was able to resist the inquisitive onslaught of the new science of objectivity and the growing belief that anything nature could do, humanity could do better. The accumulated experience of millennia was dismissed as old wives tales—the mumbo-jumbo of the past. At best it was seen as inspired guesswork and at worst as witchcraft.

THE IMPACT OF LICENSED AND PATENTED MEDICINES

In the West the decline of natural plant medicine was the quickest and most profound. One reason for this was the emergence of a system of licensed medicines linked to and protected by patents. For the first time, synthetic drugs based on specific active ingredients were developed to 'treat, cure or prevent' particular diseases. At the heart of this system lay the belief that diseases are caused by particular viruses, bacteria, fungi etc. and could be defeated by identifying and applying the appropriate anti-bacterial, antiviral, anti-fungal agent.

The safety and efficacy of these new drugs could obviously not be evaluated through traditional use, as had been the case with plant medicines for centuries. Instead an entirely new licensing system had to be created, capable of both evaluating the efficacy of these new chemical entities and assuring the public that they were safe. The licensing system devised, which still operates today, required firstly that the chemicals that made up the new drugs be always the same, in both the clinical trials undertaken to test their efficacy and in any subsequently manufactured drug. Secondly, the compounds tested had to prove through clinical trials *in vivo*, i.e. in human patients, that they were effective against specific disease conditions or disease agents and had no long-term toxic or adverse effects when used.

It did not take long to recognise that there was a price to pay for such chemical drugs. It was not always possible to identify within a short period the long-term effects of the drugs and inevitably some, perhaps most, drugs had greater or lesser short-term side effects. So another concept was developed to deal with this problem, that of risk-benefit. A drug may be shown to be immediately effective in a particular area, for example, in reducing inflammation in conditions like arthritis, yet have some unavoidable side effects in connection with the operation of some other bodily function, e.g. the stomach. Those responsible for licensing had to calculate the extent to which the benefit of the new drug balanced the risk or negative side of it. From the beginning it was possible to licence a new drug for a particular purpose even though it was known to have specific side effects.

In effect this licensing process created a new and radically different definition of medicine—one based on the specific identifiable effect of a narrow range of synthetic, replicable chemical compounds. This new category now offers the only definition of medicine, as orthodox or traditional medicine. Traditional medicines—plant-based medicines in use since time began—are now labeled 'alternative', 'complementary' or—'natural'. The inevitable connotation of these 'alternative' labels is that they are somehow inferior, ineffective or inappropriate in a modern scientific world.

Even now, as society recognises more and more the down side of this synthetic 'risk-benefit' definition of medicine, the system of licensing developed to regulate it is still seen as the only appropriate way of assuring the consumer of the safety of all medicines, synthetic and natural. The problem is that it is virtually impossible to evaluate 'natural' medicines—whole plant-based medicines—using a system created to regulate synthetic chemical drugs. To begin with, natural medicines are highly complex biochemical compounds—far more complex than synthetic drugs—containing, as in the case of propolis, hundreds of separate biochemicals. Although the rough biochemical 'fingerprint' of propolis found in different areas may remain similar, the presence and quantities of particular elements may vary enormously and are far from predictable.

Secondly, for many natural products, the Grail-like search for specific active ingredients has proved futile. Scientists are increasingly coming to realise that natural medicines work holistically and synergistically: the more complete and whole, they are the less refined and purified, the more effective they appear to be. The increasing medicinal use of St John's wort provides a good example of the problem. Recognising the value of St John's wort for treating depression, scientists believed they had found the active element in hypericin, only to find out later that hypericin itself has some significant adverse effects: it photosensitizes the skin and can increase the risk of skin cancer. New actives are now being identified and trumpeted whilst the medical herbalists wait patiently for medical science to realise that it is the effect of the whole plant extract that achieves the result.

Finally, 'natural' medicines, whilst they may have a reputation for treating a specific health problem, are often effective across a broad range of conditions rather than for one single problem. Propolis is a good example but there are many others. The assumption of 'orthodox' medicine is that drugs exist to treat single problems and that those who claim a variety of benefits for natural medicines are somehow deluded. How then can natural medicines ever be evaluated by a licensing system designed to regulate a form of medication so utterly different?

The patent system adds a final ironic twist to the reinvention and renaming of medicines. Because chemical medicines are based on single synthetic chemical entities, they can be registered as unique inventions. This means that the inventors of these drugs can prevent anyone else producing them for a fixed period of years. In one sense this system does make sense. To develop a new drug can take years and in some cases millions of pounds. It does not seem fair that the companies developing the drug should spend all the money only for others to step in and reap the benefit. However, it only makes sense if you fundamentally believe in the nature of what is being protected.

Certainly, our belief in drug-based medicine has become almost complete during this last century, so much so that we have been unwilling to recognise the mounting price that we have apparently been paying for it. Not only have vast fortunes been made out of this kind of medicine by the drug companies, but it now seems clear that we have only postponed illness rather than cured it. More frightening than this is the probability that we have created a whole new genre of health problems with our chemical treatments, problems which we go on to treat with more drugs. The ultimate hidden cost of our belief in essentially unnatural medicine is likely to be beyond our imagination in terms of the universal weakening of the immune defence mechanism of humanity worldwide.

It is hard to measure the effect which the patent system has had on the development of modern medicine. Patents have undoubtedly locked us into a synthetic drug-based system of medicine and to the same extent locked us out of the valuable contribution which whole natural products could make to maintaining good health. In the Soviet Union and in the many Eastern European countries influenced by them following the Communist revolution no patent laws existed. There was not, therefore, the same pressure to put profit before the potential of natural substances. Propolis as with other natural medicines continued to be used both as a folk medicine and to be tested by scientists.

Dr Mansfield,[1] a doctor and the first Director of the Propolis Information Bureau, puts his finger on it.

> 'Neither patents, nor chemistry need dictate our lives. In Eastern Europe patents have not been an issue, so different questions have been asked—what do we have and what can we use it for? Research Institutes in China, Russia and other former Soviet bloc countries have as a result come up with very different results from their Western counterparts. We should study their methods and results urgently, and not be too hasty to convert them to our own'.

Referring specifically to propolis, Dr Mansfield reminds us how, prior to 1993, the Western scientific community showed little or no interest in propolis despite increasing interest in popular natural health publications. When it did begin to show an interest, 'their interest is in discovering its active ingredients and isolating them as patentable medicines.'[2]

PROPOLIS IN EASTERN EUROPE

The Eastern Europeans in general and Russia in particular continued to use propolis and other natural medicines long after they had been discarded in the West. Beekeeping in Eastern European countries has always been an important agricultural activity and propolis a valued by-product of honey production. The wild bees of the Caucasus produce large quantities of propolis to help them survive the harsh continental winters. For generations local people have used propolis to treat a very wide range of health problems including coughs, colds and chest problems, burns and wounds and dental problems.

One of the most often quoted and dramatic uses of propolis occurred during the Boer War in South Africa, where it was used extensively to treat wounds. Propolis was mixed with Vaseline and the mixture, known as Propolis Vanogen, was applied in many cases following surgery, and in particular following amputations. But the Russians had been using something similar many years before, at the time of Napoleon's ill-fated invasion of that country. In Napoleon's army the traditional treatment following amputation was to tar the amputated stump, but in the Russian army the doctors instead dressed the stump, with the scrapings of the honey barrels carried with them for provisions. These dregs contained high levels of propolis and assisted rapid and complete healing.

With the birth of modern medical science at the turn of the century, Russian and Eastern European countries turned naturally to the scientific process to look again at age-old remedies. We shall see when we look in detail at the science behind propolis over the last 40 years that it is dominated by work carried out in Russia, Poland, Romania, Czechoslovakia, Bulgaria and Yugoslavia. During the Second World War, for example, Russian doctors successfully experimented with the use of propolis ointment in treating wounds at two clinics in Sverdlovsk. In 1947 the Veterinary Institute of Kazan, on the edge of the Urals, undertook one of the earliest scientific investigations into the anti-microbial properties of propolis. So successful was this work that propolis became known as Russian penicillin. Ironically, just as the West is beginning to fund research into propolis Russian research institutes are struggling following the fall of Communism.

In Yugoslavia, Mitja Vosnack,[3] one-time foreign minister of Yugoslavia, eventually left politics to pursue his interest in the honeybee and propolis. In his book *The Miracle of Propolis* he recounts the experience of a nineteenth-century Yugoslavian church painter, Rado Seifert. Seifert first started keeping bees when he received two hives as payment for a job. It was sometime afterwards that he began to have trouble with his leg. The skin on his foot turned purple and then black. He lost the feeling in his foot and an ulcer opened up which simply refused to heal. Every week he went to the doctor, who prescribed ointments, but the problem got worse. Finally, the doctor recommended amputation. Rado turned down the doctor's advice and instead went home and covered his leg with honey and propolis and bandaged the whole thing up. After a few days he removed the bandage. The ulcer was gone, the foot no longer hurt and he could stand on it. After using propolis again to help heal a burn his wife had suffered he decided it was time to tell the doctor of this wonderful new medicine. But the doctor, despite having seen Rado's leg heal, was not impressed and he refused to try it on his patients. Some time later however, a friend's daughter was suffering from chronic tonsillitis which became so bad her tonsils began to suppurate while her temperature rose to 39°C (103°F). The doctor decided to try propolis delivered on a sugar cube. Within a few hours her temperature was down and the inflammation cleared, never to return.

In 1962 Mitja Vosnack's own friend was apparently dying of cancer. His friend's physician prescribed for him 10–15 drops of propolis liquid in water three times a day, half-an-hour before meals. After six weeks he had begun to eat and gain weight and his old enthusiasm and energy began to return.[4] Propolis, says Vosnak, 'is without a past, for we are only now starting to learn about it and in learning have become convinced that in propolis we have indeed discovered the medicine of the future' Propolis, for Vosnack, is not like a normal drug; rather it is a natural supplement. 'Would you call the sun a medicine? Is forest air or fresh clear water a medicine? Is an apple?'

A REVIVAL OF INTEREST IN THE WEST

In the West we had to wait until the late 1960s and early 1970s before serious interest in propolis was rekindled. Some would argue that nothing was the same in the West after the 1960s. Certainly at that time a generation came to maturity in both Europe and America who were intent on taking a fresh look at most things. Flower power expressed a re-awakening of interest in all things natural and 'alternative'—religion, education, economics and, of course, medicine. As far as natural medicine was concerned, this was a movement pioneered essentially by lay people or self-taught practitioners as much as by doctors or scientists. They were enthusiasts, entrepreneurs, health food shopkeepers, lay practitioners and the like, who believed in the ways of nature.

In 1974 Dr K. Lund Aagard, a Danish naturalist, published *The Natural Product Propolis—the Way to Health.*[5] This book contained the results of 20 years' practical experience and research into propolis. It was a book which was to earn him the title Mr Propolis and links his name firmly with the re-discovery of propolis in the West.

As is so often the case it was a personal experience which triggered what was to become a lifetime of research. In June 1962 Aagard had been suffering from a sore throat for several days. He knew that on the following day he had to go on a business trip. By evening however, the swelling was so bad he could not swallow and he had a temperature of 40°C (104°F). He decided to try some propolis, crushed a small amount in a mortar and dissolved the powder in a cup of warm water. He filtered the liquid through a coffee filter, ending up with a yellow infusion-like tea. He gargled with this tea two or three times, then drank the rest and went to bed. In the morning he found his sore throat had completely gone. Dr Aagard drew the conclusion that 'propolis contains a very strong antibiotic if it could cure such a powerful infection and swelling in just five to six hours.'

Aagard was a practical scientist and conducted extensive research involving more than 50,000 people throughout Scandinavia as well as patenting the first process for cleaning propolis. He sums up propolis in the following way: 'Propolis is one of the most efficient bee products from the viewpoint of active principles transmitted from plant to man.'[6]

As a result of his research Aagard claims that propolis can be effective in treating a bewildering variety of problems including swelling of the large intestine, catarrh of the eyes, infection of the urinary tract, swelling of the throat, gout, open wounds, sinus swellings, colds, influenza, bronchitis, gastritis, cancer, diseases of the ears, periodontal diseases, caephalea, intestinal infections, mycoses, ulcers, eczema eruptions, pneumonia, arthritis, lung disease, stomach virus, headaches, Parkinson's disease, bile infections, sclerosis, circulation deficiencies, warts, conjunctivitis and hoarseness.[7] For those who believe medicines are designed to cure specific ailments this long list must seem like heresy.

As Dr Aagard said, propolis is an extremely effective way of delivering the benefits of the plant world to man. It does not operate in the same way as a chemical seeking out and destroying the enemy bacteria, virus or whatever but rather supports the body's own ability to fight disease. 'Propolis has a refreshing effect both for regulating hormones and as an antibiotic substance, which is in itself a stimulator of the natural resistance of the body. Propolis may be used by everybody, sick or healthy, as a means of protection against microorganisms.'[8]

A French doctor at the Sorbonne in Paris, Dr Remy Chauvin, heard of Dr Aagard's work and joined forces with him. Dr Chauvin is scarcely less enthusiastic about the potential of propolis. 'The amazing fact, however, is that bee propolis has a 100 per cent killing effect on bacteria. No other antibiotic has this total effect.'[9] Dr Chauvin believes that nature has the answer to everything and that all we have to do is find it.

> With the introduction of bee propolis, it is possible that we can one day abolish many drug-related chemicals and their

side effects. Propolis works by raising the body's natural resistance to infection through stimulating one's own immune system. In doing this, propolis also supplies added amounts of vitamins, and all essential minerals, including iron, calcium, aluminium, manganese and silicon.[10]

This, Dr Chauvin points out, is very important because synthetic antibiotics do exactly the opposite. They kill the friendly bacteria in the system, which the body uses to synthesize Vitamin B and K, causing severe deficiencies. Chauvin continues by observing what we are today being constantly reminded of, that bacteria are developing a resistance to antibiotics, causing a rise in the incidence of infections and a marked increase in the ability of these diseases to pass from one person to another. Once-minor infections are becoming potential killers.

Aagard and Chauvin have been responsible perhaps more than any others for the re-awakening of scientific interest in propolis in the West. But it took the practical entrepreneurial vision of others to bring propolis to the public.

Warren Ogren was an amateur beekeeper living in a small town in Wisconsin. In the late 1960s Warren heard about Dr Aagard and his work on propolis and was sufficiently inspired to make the trip to Denmark to see him. Dr Aagard taught Ogren how to clean and process propolis and for four years was his only customer. At that time propolis was selling for around $200 per kilo, a huge amount compared to the world market price today of around $20 per kilo.

Eventually Ogren started making up his own propolis products to sell to the public. To start with he produced propolis capsules, throat sprays and skin cream. Linda Graham, Ogren's daughter, takes up the story: 'The formulations were made by trial and error (lots of errors) in the back of our house. He gave away hundreds of free samples to friends and family those first years, just to see how the product would work. Half of our small town of Hayward has had a sample of some product my father first formulated.'[11] The company which Warren Ogren started now sells propolis all over the world.

Royden Brown,[12] from Phoenix, Arizona, became another champion of propolis. He was one of the first Americans to sign up with the Canadian Air Force in 1939, and was soon based in England, flying missions over Germany. It was in England that he first came across an article in a newspaper extolling the virtues of bee products. After the war and a successful career as a banker and entrepreneur, he turned his unique energy to health and in particular to the important role honeybee products could play in maintaining that. The company he started in 1976 is now one of the largest bee products companies in the world producing honey, royal jelly, pollen and propolis. Royden Brown was one of those people who, once they became convinced of the rightness of something, go for it 100 per cent. His book *The Worlds' Only Perfect Food* is, in his words, 'a joyous celebration of the life of *Apis mellifera*, the little critters who work so hard to provide mankind with the mysterious and powerful products of the beehive.' Royden Brown died tragically in 1989 but his company continues, run by his son Bruce Brown, who shares the same passion for the honeybee and who has built the most advanced plant in the world for refining propolis.

In the UK the herbalist and pioneer wholefood shop proprietor Ray Hill[13] was the first person to write a book about propolis. In *Propolis—The Natural Antibiotic*. He echoes the theme of this section: 'so much ancient wisdom has been lost to modern man, but fortunately this remarkable substance, put into daily use by the bees, has in recent years been ''re-discovered'' and its effectiveness is constantly being proved by scientific research.'

Dr Felix Murat,[14] an American, has encapsulated a lifetimes' interest and fascination with propolis in his comprehensive and enthusiastic book *Propolis—The Eternal Natural Healer* published in 1982. For a number of years this was one of very few books solely about propolis. It is a powerful and passionate testimony to the importance of propolis and to natural living. In 1987, Jacob Kaal,[15] a Dutch beekeeper and apitherapist, published the results of decades of research into the medicinal properties of honeybee products in his book *Natural Medicines from Honeybees*. This influential little book brought together the then contemporary research in the West illustrating the mounting interest in propolis. For Kaal, as for Aagard, 'propolis is the most effective means of applying plant-derived therapeutic substances to the human body.

While honey and pollen are often very effective against illness with non-specific symptoms, propolis can be used specifically against infections—both internal and external.'

Slowly, through the 1960s, 70s and 80s, propolis came to be recognised again as a powerful natural medicine. In 1978 Dr John Diamond,[16] President of the International Academy of Preventive Medicine, speaking of propolis, told us that of all the natural substances he had tested, 'the one that seems to be the most strengthening to the thymus, and hence the Life Energy, is bee resin, or bee propolis.'

During this period propolis products became available in the West, principally through healthfood stores, and interest grew amongst the alternative health community. But we had to wait until the late eighties and early nineties before so-called serious scientific interest emerged, with a trickle of peer-reviewed papers appearing in scientific journals in Britain, USA, France, Germany and Japan. This trickle is now turning into a flood. In 1997, Dr Paul Weightman and Carmen Garcia, of the Department of Agricultural Economics, University of Newcastle[17] set out to identify the extent of work on propolis published in scientific databases between 1980 and 1995. The table below lists approximately 350 articles in this period.

Topics covered in the research papers identified cover the composition of propolis, pharmacology, allergic reactions and clinical use.

It is interesting that between 1980 and 1995 more articles appeared in the USA than in any other country. Weightman and Garcia noted that over the fifteen year period studied there was a steady improvement in the quality of the research undertaken: 'Interest moves from folklore and commentary on traditional medicines towards the rigour of advanced scientific study.' They note that interest is no longer centred in Eastern Europe but is spreading all over the world: 'Interest in propolis is becoming more widespread, and by professional, respected scientists capable of publishing in peer review journals.'

Table 2: Published articles on propolis in scientific databases 1980–1995 (Weightman and Garcia, University of Newcastle upon Tyne, 1997).

Country	**Number of Articles**
USA	32
Bulgaria	26
Germany	29
Poland	24
Yugoslavia	22
Italy	22
USSR	21
Romania	20
Ukraine	17
France	14
Czechoslovakia	14
United Kingdom	13
Spain	13
Japan	11
Cuba	8
India	4
Brazil	4
Argentina	3
New Zealand	3
Netherlands	3
Egypt	3
Israel	3

Either one or two publications:

- Australia
- Austria
- China
- Canada
- Portugal
- Singapore
- Switzerland
- South Africa
- Zaire

CHAPTER 5

How Does Propolis Work?

We have seen that propolis fulfils a comprehensive and important role in maintaining the health of the bee colony. We have also seen in our panoramic sketch of the history of its traditional use by man as a medicine that it has had a wide range of powerful and medicinal uses. It's time now to ask how it works. What is it in propolis that does the business?

In modern pharmacology we are used to asking this question and getting a reasonably straightforward answer. It is the complex action of a limited number of active ingredients or elements within the product, sometimes even just the one. Modern medicine has been dominated by our search for so-called active ingredients—those specific, unique and hopefully patentable biochemicals which hold the key to the destruction of a particular microbe, virus or fungus. Modern drug-based medicine invokes a reductionist mind-set which believes it can pin every element down as having a specific identifiable function rather than a belief in and understanding of the way whole products operate synergistically. By understanding the separate parts it is believed we can replicate them, take out the bits we want and throw away those we don't need. Rudolf Steiner,[1] a natural scientist at the turn of the century, grasped the way modern science was going at an early stage of its development.

> A pupil of the famous Bunge, the Professor of Physiology, made experiments in feeding mice with milk. The mice had a good time of it; they throve extremely well when they were fed on milk. So now he made the experiment in another way. He said to himself: the mice throve splendidly on milk; milk consists of casein, fat, sugar and salts. Consequently I shall

give some mice casein, fat, sugar and salts; . . . And behold! When he gave the mice casein, fat, sugar and salt they died within a few days. They got the same things but they all died.

Dr Peter Mansfield,[2] the founder of Good Health Keeping, has worked most of his life as a general practitioner in England. Disenchanted with what he sees as an obsession with negative health, i.e. concern only with dealing with ill-health, he now runs a natural alternative to the National Health Service, in Louth in Lincolnshire. Seventy years after Rudolf Steiner's observation he makes a similar observation.

'The fact is Western therapeutics is driven by the need to discover more and more patentable new chemicals, each of which gives its inventor a head start over its rivals. Natural medicines are out, however cheap and effective they are, they cannot be patented. So companies are driven to dissect natural products looking for an ingredient for a purification method they can make their own.'

Referring specifically to propolis he says:

It is unlikely that such an analytical approach will ever prove successful . . . analysis of this material yields a plethora of aromatic organic compounds and bioflavonoids in varying concentrations, none of which individually appears to be the *essential ingredient* (my emphasis). To the altruistic scientist this does not much matter; he is happy to work with a crude alcoholic extract of the whole propolis material. But it frustrates the hunt for patents.

Some of its properties defy not just chemical analysis but the very principles of chemistry. The interior of the beehive is a remarkably clean, sterile place—far more so than the surgical departments of hospitals. Yet this is achieved not by dosing all the bees individually, nor by lining the entire honey comb, but by an outer skin of propolis alone.

WHAT IS IN PROPOLIS?

Personal research at the International Bee Research Institute in Cardiff, turned up 52 research papers produced between 1973 and 1994 exploring the chemical constituents of propolis and a further 600+ exploring the many-sided properties of propolis. Propolis contains some 150 different biochemical entities and more are being discovered every year. The chemical composition of propolis will vary according to the local flora, the climatic zone, and the type of bees collecting it, the season it is collected in and even the time of day it is collected. I am not a scientist, let alone a pharmacologist, but it is clear to me reading these papers that we have only just begun to understand the operation of some of the principal groups of elements in the propolis collected in mainly temperate climatic zones. Propolis collected in tropical zones contains sometimes radically different concentrations of biochemicals and yet still has a range of similar pharmacological properties.

If we are still not sure what is in propolis, how can we expect to understand what some 150 individual biochemicals are doing, let alone how those biochemicals are acting synergistically? This is not an argument for not doing the science; rather, it is an argument for humility and for not rejecting something because we do not know exactly how it works. It is in this context that we turn to exploring those groups of elements and single elements, which have emerged as playing a crucial pharmacological role in relation to particular medicinal properties of propolis. Broadly speaking these fall into four groups.[3]

Beeswax constituents

These are principally esters of fatty acids and long chain hydrocarbon alcohols which are largely inactive chemically although extensively used in cosmetics. However, where propolis is used medicinally it is often in an extract from which the beeswax has been removed.

Volatile constituents

The characteristic aroma of propolis is due mainly to these substances, mainly terpenes, although propolis found in temperate zones contains comparatively small amounts of them and very little is known about their biological activity. Propolis in tropical zones however contains far more and are known to have significant biological activity.

Phenolic compounds

These include caffeic acid phenylethylester or CAPE which research has shown to produce some of the medicinal properties.[4]

Flavonoids

These are found in nearly all flowering plant species. Dozens of these have been isolated in propolis, of which pinocembrin and galangin are thought to be most important. It is interesting to note, however, that flavonoids in plants show subtle biochemical changes when they appear in propolis, which is thought to be as a result of the enzymic action of the bee's salivary glands. Flavonoid content in propolis can range from 10–20 per cent and form the largest single biochemical group within propolis. It is the flavonoid content of propolis, which has given rise to the most concerted interest on the part of researchers.

Flavonoids in European propolis can comprise up to 20 per cent of its weight. There is a major difference between the flavonoids found in plants and those found in propolis. Those found in propolis are not glycosides, that is. They do not have sugars attached to their biochemical structure as those found in plants do. The difference may well be due to the way the bee 'process' these flavonoids through the secretion of enzymes. The fact is, they are changed, and this may well explain some of the unique therapeutic qualities of propolis.

There has been some debate concerning the presence of flavonoids in other products from the beehive i.e. in the pollen and honey. Sabatier and others conducted some research at the

University of Coimbra, Portugal, in 1995 and found that the total flavonoid content in pollen was 0.5 per cent, honey 0.006 per cent and in propolis 10 per cent.

THE ROLE OF BIOFLAVONOIDS

Bioflavonoids have created considerable interest worldwide over the last twenty years. In 1974 naturopathic physician Paavo Airola,[5] was able to claim that 'over five hundred scientific papers on bioflavonoids have been published in reputable medical journals around the world. Clinical reports have shown that bioflavonoid therapy is effective in such diversified conditions as rheumatic fever, spontaneous abortions and miscarriages, high blood pressure, respiratory infections, haemorrhoids, cirrhosis of the liver.'[6] By the 1990s scientific interest had increased dramatically.

Carlson Wade,[7] in his excellent introduction to propolis, *Propolis: Nature's Energizer* published the details of a personal interview with Bent Havsteen MD of Kiel University, who has published extensively on the importance of flavonoids in propolis. This interview provides some clear and dramatic insight into the role of bioflavonoids and through it the dynamic role of propolis as a whole.

> Bioflavonoids in propolis have a protective effect on virus infections. Let me explain. Viruses are enclosed in a protein coat. As long as it remains unbroken, the infectious and dangerous material remains imprisoned and is harmless to the organism. We have found that an enzyme, which normally removes the protein coat, is being inhibited; thus, dangerous viral material is kept locked in. The protein coating around the virus is maintained by the bioflavonoids in propolis; these flavonoids keep the virus inactive. It is the same as being immune to the virus but only with the presence of bioflavonoids as in the propolis.

This provides us with a fascinating and graphic illustration of the role of flavonoids in propolis. When I first read it in 1992 it reminded me vividly of the way in the bees themselves deal with intruders into the hive. They surround and seal up the source of infection with propolis in just the same way as the bioflavonoids seal in the virus, preventing it from entering into the body. In this way we see that the virus, rather than being destroyed, is disabled, a process which also strikes me as a metaphor for the difference between natural and allopathic medicine. Natural (whole) medicine is about working with and maintaining the ecology and balance of the body, rather than destroying diseases. A strong immune system is one where the creative and destructive forces are kept in balance, not where one element must defeat the other.

Dr Havsteen continues: 'The action of propolis bioflavonoids is almost identical with that of aspirin. They block the same enzyme. But propolis has an advantage over aspirin because it has no side effects.' For example, in the case of sore throats caused by inflamed and infected mucous membrane, 'the bioflavonoids in propolis actually block the building of prostaglandins (which cause the pain). It is like building immunity to sore throats and related winter ailments.'[8] Sticking with the theme of immunity, Dr Havsteen tells us that bioflavonoids stimulate the white bloods cells and lymphocytes into producing interferon the natural protein substance now recognised as central to a healthy immune system.

Bioflavonoids work the same way in preventing allergies.

> Histamine and serotonin are tissue hormones. They remain in the master cells. But when an allergen binds itself to the outside of the cell, these two substances leak out and cause an allergic reaction. The trick is to block the leakage of these substances. We have found that this can be done with the use of bioflavonoids in propolis. They block the acids that would break into the cells and cause the release of the allergy-causing substances. Again we see that propolis can create this form of built-in immunity.

Once again the image is of a substance strengthening a natural balance rather than destroying or removing any single element.

Finally, Havsteen provides us with some insight into an area we will look at later, that is the role of propolis in treating dental problems, in particular those caused by inflammation of the gums, mouth ulcers and erosion and infectious bleeding of the gums and tissues that line the mouth. As we have seen, the bioflavonoids in propolis block the production of prostaglandins which cause decomposition. 'But there is another benefit. The bioflavonoids stimulated enzyme formation to fortify the walls of the blood vessels in the gums. In this way, we have a two-pronged or multi-pronged attack on the diseased area of the mouth.'

The key words here are blocking, sealing in, locking in, fortifying and building up. Bioflavonoids appear to have a general protective function within the body. Perhaps more than any other factor this explains the incredible range of properties possessed by propolis, properties we have come to recognise only as single specific pharmacological effects: antibiotic, anti-inflammatory, anti-fungal, etc. Our imaginations rebel against the idea of a single product, which wraps all these functions into one. But should it? Perhaps what we have done with 'active ingredient medicine' is to identify only the fighting force against disease, the armed element, and forget the diplomats, the field surgeons, and the myriad of other hidden elements that go into finding a long-lasting and whole solution.

PHARMACOLOGICAL RESEARCH

The following pharmacological properties have been attributed to propolis in research carried out over the last 30 years.

- anaesthetic/analgesic
- anti-allergen
- antacid
- antibiotic
- anti-fungal
- anti-inflammatory
- anti-radiation
- antioxidant and preservative
- antiseptic
- anti-tumour/cancer
- antiviral and immuno-stimulant effects.

Anaesthetic/analgesic

This is one of the most intriguing and least understood properties of propolis. Anyone who chews good quality raw propolis for any period will soon recognise the numbing effect it produces in the mouth; it even has an anaesthetic-like smell. Propolis has traditionally been used to reduce pain externally in wounds, burns and especially mouth ulcers. Awareness of this characteristic no doubt encouraged researchers to explore its use as an anaesthetic.

In 1957 the Russian researcher, Prokopovich[9] and others found that an alcoholic extract of propolis produced an anaesthetic effect on rabbit cornea that they believed to be stronger than that of cocaine or procaine. Similar experiments were repeated at the Veterinary Institute of Bulgaria by Tsakov[10] in 1973. These confirmed a similar anaesthetic effect using ethanolic and aqueous extracts of propolis but much weaker—30 per cent weaker than 50 per cent novocaine—than that claimed by the Russians. Two years later the same researcher[11] found that a 30 per cent ethanolic extract of propolis introduced orally produced a good anaesthetic reaction in dogs and sheep within 15–20 minutes. Tsakov claims he 'saw no difference between the anaesthetic effect and that of novocaine.'

In 1979 German researchers[12] found that ethanolic extracts of propolis and, in particular, of some of the flavonoids in propolis, notably pinocembrin, pinostrobin and caffeic acid esters each produced local anaesthetic effects on rabbit and mouse cornea. The three flavonoids, when applied alone, were found to be nearly three times as potent as the total extract. In particular, the local anaesthetic activity of pinocembrin or caffeic acid ester mixture was about one tenth of that of lidocaine.

Anti-allergen

In our earlier discussion on the role of bioflavonoids, Havsteen[13] showed how bioflavonoids operate to block an allergic reaction caused by the release of histamine and serotonin from the master cells once allergens have attached themselves. They do this by inhibiting the operation of the acids which break into the cells. However, the only known side effect of any consequence experienced by propolis users is that of allergic response. This usually manifests itself as a mild rash on contact with propolis and affects about one in 1000.

Antacid

Russian researchers in 1973[14] noted that an ethyl alcohol extract of propolis was able to reduce the acid content in pork fat.

Antibiotic

The antibiotic properties of propolis are perhaps best known and most widely researched. Sixty-seven research papers in this area alone were published between 1973 and 1994.[15] But research into the anti-microbial properties of propolis began even earlier, back in 1947 at the Kazan Veterinary Institute in the USSR. Russian work dominates the early research, illustrating why propolis came to be known as 'Russian penicillin'. What follows is a chronological cross-section of the research exploring this important property.

At the 1958 International Beekeeping Congress, Feuereisl and others[16] reported on the effectiveness of propolis against the tuberculosis bacilli (*Mycobacterium*). Tuberculosis was a serious problem in the USSR earlier in the century. Many thought it to be one of the diseases banished by modern antibiotic drugs. The re-emergence of tuberculosis worldwide, including in the UK, has revealed a strain untreatable by virtually all known antibiotics. It may be that propolis has a role to play here.

In 1960 French researchers[17] demonstrated the bacteriostatic effect of propolis on *Bacillus subtilis*, *Proteus vulgaris* and *Bacillus alvei*. The effect was less marked for *Salmonella* and *E.coli*. Still in France, at the Institute Pasteur in 1964,[18] the flavonoids galangin and pinocembrin were identified as having the strongest anti-bacterial effects.

In 1973 two Russians at the Kazan Veterinary Institute[19] published a remarkable piece of work. In earlier research, Kivalkina had illustrated the anti-microbial properties of propolis and now wanted to find out what effect the addition of propolis would have on the effectiveness of antibiotics against *Staphylococcus aureus* and *E.coli*. The results were startling. Propolis increased the bacteriostatic activity of three antibiotics, tetracycline, neomycin and polymyxin, against *Staphylococcus aureus* by between ten and 100 times. The effectiveness of a further range of antibiotics including penicillin against *E.coli* was similarly improved. They then tested the effectiveness of two antibiotic ointments when propolis was added. With propolis the ointments' bacteriostatic action commenced within 15–30 minutes whereas without propolis bacteriostatic activity took between two and 12 hours to engage. This is an area that must be worth further investigation. There is a clear potential here for both reducing the dosage of traditional antibiotics and perhaps reducing the side effects of antibiotics.

Polish scientists in 1977[20] found that the anti-bacterial effect of propolis against *Staphylococcus aureus* was only present when propolis was delivered in the whole product rather than via specific 'active' elements, i.e. particular flavonoids. In later research they found that propolis was active against only some of the *Staphylococcus* strains when isolated from pathological material. Norwegian research in 1977[21] found that propolis was not as effective against gram-positive bacteria like *Listeria monocytogenes*.

In a comprehensive study carried out in West Germany in 1979[22] propolis was compared to a range of conventional antibiotics. Propolis showed good results against some organisms but was less effective than traditional antibiotics against *Bacillus subtilis*, *Staphylococcus aureus* and *Candida albicans*.

Research was commissioned by the Russian Ministry of Health (Drugs Standards Control) in 1981[23] to test propolis against 106 different strains of *Staphylococcus aureus*. Strains resistant to some antibiotics were found to be sensitive to propolis and propolis was found to have a synergistic effect with all the antibiotics used.

Yugoslavian research conducted in 1985[24] tested 38 samples of propolis collected from all over the former Yugoslavia. Where high concentrations of the flavonoid pinocembrin were found, and less so with galangin, the greatest activity against *Bacillus subtilis* was demonstrated.

In 1986 Polish researchers[25] tested a mixture of 10 per cent ethanolic extract of propolis and 13 typical antibiotics against *Staphylococcus aureus* isolated from abscesses showing resistance to antibiotics. A compound effect was shown in 69 per cent whilst 11 per cent showed a synergistic effect.

In the same year, across the border in Czechoslovakia,[26] researchers were demonstrating how propolis appeared to inhibit the syntheses of proteins by bacteria, suggesting that this may account for its anti-microbial action. We are reminded here of Dr Bent Havsteen's research in Germany which showed how flavonoids prevent the breakdown of the protein coating of viruses by inhibiting enzymatic action thus preventing them leaking into, and 'infecting' the organism.

1987 saw American researcher Lindenfelser[27] show that propolis was active against 25 of 39 bacterial species.

Professor Scheller,[28] of the Silesian School of Medicine in Poland, has explored many aspects of propolis. In 1988 he found that an ethanolic extract of propolis (EEP) was capable of increasing the number of plaque-forming cells in the spleen cells of immunised male mice, demonstrating their ability to produce anti-bodies. The effect of the propolis was three times greater than in the controls. This effect increased if the dose was repeated and if the dose was increased.

In 1989, Cora Rosenthal,[29] an Israeli researcher, found whilst an aqueous extract of propolis had no anti-microbial effect, an ethanolic extract had an inhibitory effect on a range of bacteria including *Staphylococcus aureus*.

In 1990 Grange and Davey at the National Heart and Lung Institute, London[30] published what has turned out to be a landmark piece of research for propolis in the West. They found that in dilutions of 1:20, propolis completely inhibited the growth of *Staphylococcus aureus* including the MRSA [Methicillin Resistant Staphylococcus Aureus] strains. It partially inhibited growth of others but had no effect on still other strains. This research was important for two reasons. Firstly, it finally gave some credibility in the West to the work which had been going on in Eastern Europe for decades. Secondly, by demonstrating that propolis could inhibit MRSA it showed that propolis may have a role in helping to solve a serious and urgent problem in UK hospitals. In 1990 perhaps 50 per cent of UK hospitals were infected with MRSA. Today it is nearer 70 per cent and we still have no solution.

Back in Russia, in 1991,[31] researchers found that propolis was effective against a further range of bacteria—*Staphylococcus viridians* and *S. pyogenes*, *Diplococcus pneumonia* and the gram-negative organisms *E.coli, Salmonella spp.* and *Shigella flexneri.*

Research at the University of Ferrara, in Italy,[32] tested a range of commercial extracts of propolis for their anti-microbial and antifungal properties. The research showed that 30 per cent extracts of propolis in oil, ethanol, propylene glycol and glycerine had differing anti-microbial effects. The extracts prepared in glycerine inhibited microbial development for only a few days, whereas the other preparations maintained an inhibition for up to two weeks.

In 1996 I commissioned research at the University of Oxford. Using a commercially available alcohol propolis tincture. Dr Philip Calder and others[33] (including O. K. Mirzoeva, from the University of Moscow) explored its effect on the growth and motility of bacteria. They found that propolis was effective against gram-positive and some gram-negative bacteria. More interestingly, they found that some of the components of propolis—cinnammic acids and flavonoids in particular—had the effect of 'uncoupling' the energy field of the bacteria, inhibiting their ability to move around. They believed that this change in the bioenergetic status of the bacteria could be responsible for the anti-microbial action as well as for the way propolis works synergistically with antibiotics.

The 25 research projects listed above span a period of 40 years. Western interest has appeared in the last ten years with five out of the seven most recent studies coming from the West. Whilst some new developments have emerged from this work, in the main they confirm the findings of earlier Eastern European studies. Inevitably, results from these studies are not always consistent. Some studies emphasise the importance of the type of extract used and the amount used, others the area from which it is collected or the season in which it is collected. What we must continually bear in mind is the absence of any single standard material. Grange, in his paper, refers to propolis as an unstable substance. Perhaps complex and unpredictable would be a more appropriate description. Certainly it is impossible to truly compare research findings unless we are first and foremost clear about what material we are comparing.

Anti-fungal

Fungal problems have grown exponentially over the last ten years. Treatment with chemical drugs is increasingly difficult. The same thing has happened with anti-fungal drugs as happened with antibiotics—the fungi have learnt to adapt to and resist increasingly sophisticated and stronger chemical drugs. The new drugs are themselves now causing complex adverse reactions in the body, particularly in relation to our immune response mechanisms.

In 1973 Czechoslovak researchers[34] found that propolis was as effective against 12 micro-organisms as 12 units of penicillium or 25 units of fungicidin. Again, Czech researchers in 1975[35] showed that an ethanolic extract of propolis inhibited the growth of 60 strains of yeast tested. One year later, the same researchers[36] found that propolis had a similarly inhibitory effect on 38 strains of fungi including *Candida albicans* as well as those fungal organisms responsible for ringworm and tinea.

In 1977 Polish researchers[37] found that an ethanolic extract of propolis was lethal against the protozoa *Trichomonas vaginalis* and *Toxoplasma gondii*. This research supports research illustrating the effectiveness of propolis in treating purulent vaginal infections.

In 1979 researchers in the Federal German Republic[38] found that the flavonoid pinocembrin, present in propolis, was particularly effective against fungal infections externally, but it was not effective when injected into infected mice. Too much of the pinocembrin was excreted, leaving insufficient in the blood serum to destroy the fungi.

Research at the University of Zagreb[39] in 1982 showed that high concentrations of propolis inhibited the growth of the respiratory tract fungus *Aspergillus sulphureus* and reduced the toxins produced by it for up to ten days.

Polish researchers as the Institute of Medicinal Plants in 1987[40] tested the effect of a mixture of 10 per cent EEP and ten anti-fungal preparations on nine strains of *Candida albicans* isolated from human skin or the mucous membrane. They found that propolis improved the effectiveness of all the preparations but worked most effectively when combined with natamycin and flucytosine.

In 1987 Cuban researchers[41] tested aqueous and alcoholic extracts of propolis against two strains of *Candida albicans*. The aqueous extract had no effect and the alcoholic extract had only a weak effect. French research in the same year[42] compared the effectiveness of propolis with nine anti-fungal drugs on four fungi that cause infections in humans. Propolis was as effective or more effective than most of the other preparations against three of the fungi. The most effective results were achieved against *Scopulariopsis brevicaulis* using a combination of propolis with propylene glycol. Propylene glycol appeared to enhance the effectiveness of propolis all round.

Finally, in 1989 Czech researchers[43] tested a 10 per cent ethanolic extract of propolis against 17 fungal pathogens. Propolis was found to be active against them all. Of seven components of propolis separately tested, benzoic acid, salicyclic acid and vanillin were identified as strongly fungistatic.

Anti-inflammatory

The inflammatory response occurs when cell membranes are ruptured and fatty acids are produced, which in turn produce arachidonic acid, triggering the creation of prostaglandins and leukotrienes. The prostaglandins and leukotrienes cause leakage from blood capillaries—reddening of skin tissue, release of histamine, pain and a collection of fluid in the area.

Ruptured cell membranes
LEAD TO
Release of fatty acids
LEAD TO
Production of arachidonic acid
LEAD TO
Production of prostaglandins and leukotrienes
WHICH CAUSE
Leakage from blood capillaries
Reddening of the skin
Release of histamine
Pain and collection of fluid

Diagram 1: The inflamatory process

The inflammatory process is a key factor in a variety of debilitating diseases including asthma, psoriasis, adult respiratory distress syndrome, allergic rhinitis, gout, rheumatoid arthritis, migraines, inflammatory bowel disease, gingivitis and mouth ulceration.

In a study of propolis consumers carried out in 1995 nearly 70 per cent were using it to treat health problems caused by inflammation. Thirty-nine per cent used it for arthritis, rheumatism and muscular pain, 18 per cent used it for asthma and bronchitis, and ten per cent used it for skin problems like eczema and psoriasis.

We have already examined Dr Bent Havsteen's research at the University of Keil in 1978. In that work he showed how he believed that flavonoids blocked the enzymes seeking to rupture the cell membrane thus, preventing the inflammatory process from starting.[44]

In 1979 a Romanian patent[45] was registered for a product containing propolis and described as having anti-inflammatory and antiseptic properties. The product was to be delivered as a gel for application to inflamed mucosal conditions. Researchers in Romania in 1984[46] induced rheumatic fever in rats and then fed them propolis extract daily. The treatment led to a remission of the symptoms of the fever including a softening of the cartilage around the joints and a reduction of lesions.

Hungarian researchers reporting to the International Congress of Apiculture in Japan in 1986[47] showed how certain fractions and isolated compounds of propolis and a commercially available product reduced inflammation when fed to rats with induced inflammatory conditions.

In 1996 a unique collaborative research venture between the Silesian Medical School, the National Institute of Health in Japan and the Hebrew University, Jerusalem,[48] reported its findings. Various isolated phenolic components of propolis were tested for their degree of anti-inflammatory activity. CAPE (caffeic acid phenylethyl ester) was found to be 100 per cent effective using the method chosen whilst the three flavonoids (galangin, kaempferol and kaempferid) were 73–93 per cent effective.

In the same year research commissioned by the author took place at the University of Oxford.[49] Propolis and various components of propolis, notably CAPE, were tested for their anti-inflammatory effect on acute peritoneal inflammation *in vivo* (mice). Dietary propolis significantly suppressed the creation of arachidonic acid which leads on to creation of prostaglandins. However, CAPE was most effective in blocking the development of prostaglandins.

The last two pieces of research provide powerful evidence of the ability of propolis, and in particular of certain components of propolis, to inhibit the inflammatory process. Problems in the West with anti-inflammatory drugs reflect the nature and scale of problems with antibiotics and anti-fungal drugs. In particular, the tendency of some commonly used drugs to cause serious damage to the stomach has caused alarm amongst users. The prospect of developing a natural alternative in this huge market has no doubt encouraged researchers.

Anti-irradiation

Strictly speaking, the remarkable piece of research discussed below belongs to the above section. Radiation is a significant stimulant for free radicals. In a nuclear age we are surrounded not only by the dangerous potential of nuclear power and nuclear weapons but also are continually over-exposed to low-level radiation through X-rays and other forms.

In 1989[50] researchers at Silesian School of Medicine in Poland, and the University of Southern California, collaborated in a project designed to test the extent to which propolis could protect mice exposed to gamma radiation. One group of mice was injected with a propolis preparation both before and after the gamma irradiation. The second group was not treated at all. The non-treated mice died within 12 weeks whereas the mice treated with propolis survived. In the surviving group the leucocyte count as well as their spleen plaque formation activity returned to normal. The authors suggest that an antioxidant and free radical scavenger in the propolis was responsible for the protective effect. Protection is greatest if the propolis is delivered prior to or shortly after the irradiation.

Antioxidant and preservative

The natural process of breakdown that goes on continually in the body leads to the production of so-called free radicals. These free oxygen molecules would, if not mopped up and balanced by the production of antioxidants, lead inevitably to the complete breakdown of the organism through cancer, heart disease, arthritis and a variety of other degenerative diseases. Stress, infections, X-rays, pollution and poor diet all contribute to the creation of free radicals. Interest in understanding and managing antioxidant activity has been very high over recent years. The review of research which follows looks at the role of propolis as a preservative as well as ways in which propolis can assist living organisms to maintain the free radical–antioxidant balance.

PROPOLIS AS A PRESERVATIVE

In 1976 researchers at the Russian National Bee Keeping Institute, Ryazan,[51] found that an extract of propolis had more than twice the antioxidant activity of synthetic preservatives when applied to ground white fish stored in a refrigerator.

Similar research was conducted by the Egyptian Ministry of Agriculture in 1980.[52] Five natural substances, including an ethanolic extract of propolis, were tested as antioxidants in frozen meat. The aqueous extract was found to have less effect than the ethanolic extract, which was found to have the greatest effect of all the compounds tested. Interestingly, bearing in mind the powerful taste and smell of propolis, the flavour of the meat was unaffected.

In 1980 the Institute of Veterinary Medicine, Belgrade,[53] tested six different propolis extracts on fresh lard at 10°C (50°F). Propolis and all its extracts had strong antioxidant effects, though there were some differences between the extracts. Similar research was undertaken at the Department of Veterinary Medicine in Belgrade in 1981.[54] The antioxidant/preservative properties of 0.1 per cent propolis solution were compared with chemical preservatives on pigs' back fat and lard samples. The propolis products were found to be equally as effective as the synthetic products.

In 1982 Veterinary researchers in Belgrade[55] again used propolis dissolved in 96 per cent ethanol to preserve anatomical specimens of muscle, liver, kidney and other tissues. After six months the samples were still in good condition.

Bulgarian researchers in 1984[56] chose to test the extent to which 1–5 per cent concentrations of propolis would prevent oxidation in lard (chosen as a model lipid system). They looked at both the effect of propolis as a whole and at the action of individual flavonoids. They found that best results were achieved using the whole propolis extract and that individual flavonoids were not as effective.

The commercial potential of using propolis as a preservative for food is recognised by two Japanese patents, one for a propolis product that can be applied to the food itself[57] and another where propolis is integrated into food packaging.[58]

ANTIOXIDANT EFFECTS IN LIVE ORGANISMS

Russian researchers at the Alma Ata Medical Institute in 1986[59] found that propolis fed to mice with salmonella stabilised the lipid peroxidation caused by the disease. Propolis acted as an antioxidant and subsequent dissection showed that the extent of pathological changes usual in salmonella was much reduced. The researchers believed that propolis could provide a natural treatment for salmonella.

Two years later, in 1988, the same researchers[60] compared propolis and vitamin E as natural antioxidants. Polyunsaturated fatty acids included in animal feed increased the rate of lipid peroxidation in the animals fed. Both vitamin E and propolis stabilised this process but the increase in body weight of the animals taking propolis indicated that propolis had a stronger antioxidant effect.

In 1990 the first research in this area in the West was undertaken at the University of Southern California.[61] Their findings linked the antioxidant properties in propolis to the high quantities of flavonoids present in the extract. The propolis extract inhibited luminol H^2O^2 chemiluminescence *in vitro*.

Romanian research in 1991[62] showed that a purified water-soluble extract of propolis had an antioxidant effect on a range of chemical reactions which produce hydrogen peroxide.

Research at the Institute of Experimental Apiculture in Cuba in 1993[63] indicated that extracts of Cuban propolis had antioxidant properties and this could be attributed to their free radical scavenging activity against alkoxy radicals and, to a lesser degree, against superoxide.

Water-extracted propolis was compared with an ethanol extract in research at the University of Munich, 1993.[64] The aqueous extract of propolis was found to exhibit a higher antioxidant property and inhibitory activity than the ethanolic extracts.

In 1997, Lithuanian researchers[65] reported on their work to further test the antioxidant and pro-oxidant activity of propolis on blood lipoproteins. They found that propolis acted as an antioxidant at lower concentrations whilst at higher concentrations propolis became a pro-oxidant. Finally, work undertaken at the University of Moscow in 1994[66] showed how certain extracted compounds of propolis, notably CAPE, could block the formation of reactive oxygen species in human neutrophils.

Degenerative diseases are increasing. As we enter a new millennium four out of ten people are expected to suffer from cancer at some point in their lives and this figure is increasing. Environmental pollution and poor nutrition all make us more vulnerable. The fact that propolis operates as an antioxidant adds still greater value to it for maintaining positive health. Research illustrating the preservative properties of propolis may also begin to attract commercial interest as the public turns away from chemical and irradiation preservation systems.

Antiseptic

The effect of propolis in the hive is often referred to as antiseptic although this probably oversimplifies the effect. The most interesting research in this area was carried out in Italy in 1989. Panizzi[67] prepared a solution of two per cent propolis and 0.4 per cent essential oils in propylene glycol. He then sprayed this solution in aerosol form into three enclosed public areas—a school hall, analytical laboratory and a library. This propolis spray was found to reduce the number of microorganisms in the air by 93 per cent. Further tests would need to be done but there would seem to be a potential here for use in hospitals, particularly as part of the fight against the airborne transmission of antibiotic-resistant bacteria.

Anti-tumour/cancer

Earlier we saw anecdotal evidence of successful treatment of cancer with propolis. The pharmacological research available is modest but relatively recent. In 1988, at the Institute of Cancer Research, University of New York, USA, Grunberger[68] and his colleagues looked at the effectiveness of CAPE in an extract isolated from Israeli propolis. CAPE showed cytostatic effects on all type of cells but showed particular sensitivity to human cells. This research has created excitement amongst cancer researchers because CAPE is an easily extractable and replicable compound based on propolis.

In the same year, in the Federal Republic of Germany, Konig[69] and others reviewed the anti-cancer and antiviral properties of CAPE. They confirmed the cytostatic activity of the compound and put forward an explanation of the mechanism for its activity.

In 1989 a joint University of California-Silesian School of Medicine study[70] compared the effectiveness of EEP with the cancer drug bleomycin on mice infected with Erlich Carcinoma. It was found that the survival rate of the mice after 55 days was 50 per cent for the group treated with propolis and 44 per cent for those treated with bleomycin. The research concluded that 'the anti-tumoral property of EEP in the tumoured animal model studies is significant and lasting.'

In 1990, at the University of Cardiff, Peter Ross[71] tested various aqueous and alcoholic extracts of propolis against cancer cells and against various bacteria and fungi. All extracts were found to have limited *in vitro* cytotoxic and cytostatic effects against certain cancer cells. Propolis extracts also slowed down the development of tumours in cancer-infected mice.

Japanese research in 1992 at the National Institute of Health, Tokyo,[72] found that extracts and fractions of Brazilian propolis had a limited cytotoxic effect on cancer cells, arresting tumour development at certain stages, but had little effect on human diploid cells.

Basic and others[73] in Croatia reported their findings on the use of some propolis derivatives (CAPE) in the proceedings of the International Congress of Apiculture, 1997. The number of infected tumours in the lungs of infected mice were reduced both by preventative and curative therapy with CAPE but less so with caffeic acid only.

Much of this anti-cancer research has focused on an attempt to utilise a narrow range of components in propolis (CAPE). Understandably, this is an area where the world is looking for new life-saving drugs—drugs that make an immediate and dramatic difference. Again and again, however, we have observed that propolis is as much as a preventative as a pure treatment of disease. CAPE is perhaps the nearest candidate so far for a traditional licensed drug. It has a level of effectiveness and it can be synthesised. Unfortunately, its effect is not sufficiently dramatic to warrant the cost involved in converting it into a traditional licensed medicine.

Antiviral and immuno-stimulant effects

Viral diseases are the most difficult to control as antibiotics are not effective against them and they show a remarkable ability to change and adapt to drugs used against them.

An early study carried out by Kivalkina[74] in 1969 at the Kazan Veterinary Institute, showed that propolis had immune stimulant properties in guinea pigs infected with influenza. In 1971, Dunyavin[75] in the USSR, tested propolis and copper cobalt IKP separately in combination with a paratyphoid antigen by injection in bulls. The results showed that both propolis and copper cobalt activated production of antibodies and phagacytosis, improving immunogenesis.

In 1971 Shevchenko and others[76] in the USSR, gave a five per cent alcoholic extract of propolis solution intra-nasally or as an aerosol, to mice just two hours before they were infected with influenza. The propolis preparation completely inhibited influenza virus proliferation. Interestingly, the preparation had no effect when given to mice already infected.

In 1976 research at the Kazan Veterinary Institute[77] using aqueous and alcoholic extracts of propolis found that propolis inhibited the multiplication of the virus responsible for Aujeszky's disease, which causes paralysis in cattle, horses and pigs. Propolis was more effective with mild infections. Similar research the following year at the Institute[78] tested live Aujeszky's disease vaccine with and without propolis. Those treated with the vaccine increased their antibody formation by two–three times. The propolis treatment also enhanced production of plasmacytes in the lymphoidal tissue of the spleen and lymph nodes.

Romanian research in 1981[79] tested propolis on mice both before and after they had been infected with influenza. Unlike the earlier study, the mice fed propolis after infection lived longer than those treated prior to infection.

Another Romanian study in 1983[80] showed that rats fed with a mixture of standardized propolis extract and *E.coli* antigen showed a marked increase in the formation of antibodies compared with the group not fed on propolis.

In 1985 Konig and others[81] in the German Federal Republic, examined the role of propolis and some of its derivatives against the avian herpes virus. They tested a variety of separate compounds in propolis, including a range of flavonoids and cinnamic acid compounds. Several of the compounds related to caffeic acid produced antiviral activity, whilst several other separate cinnamic acid derivatives and flavonoids did not. In 1986 the same researchers tested a variety of extracts from tropical and non-tropical propolis samples against avian herpes and Aujeszky's virus.[82] All the samples of non-tropical propolis showed inhibition of several herpes and Aujeszky's viruses. Several caffeolic compounds showed high antiviral activity. The results indicate that the mechanism of inhibition may be related to virus-specific nucleic acid or protein synthesis. Various fractions of propolis were found to have a pronounced stimulating effect on the cell-mediated immune response in mice. In an immunobiological test there was an increase in the number of antigen-reacting cells.

In 1988 Neychev,[83] a Bulgarian researcher produced a water-soluble fraction of propolis—mainly phenol derivatives. This was found to have immunostimulant activity in mice infected with influenza type A. Mortality in the untreated mice was 100 per cent whereas in the treated mice it was 60 per cent for those treated orally, but only 40 per cent for those injected.

In 1988 Scheller and his colleagues[84] at the Silesian Medical School, tested the effect of a propolis extract administered to mice prior to immunisation. He found that the number of plague-forming cells (cells producing antibodies) in the spleen increased to three times greater than in the controls. Researchers concluded that immunisation should be carried out within 48 hours of EEP injections.

Italian researchers in 1990 tested a range of specific flavonoids on a range of viruses—herpes, adenocrona and rotavirus. Whilst quercetin showed some inhibitory effect, this was only at very high doses. The other flavonoids showed only a poor inhibitory effect.[85]

However, research undertaken by Amoros[86] at the Faculty of Pharmacy in Rennes, France, in 1992 contradicts the above findings. Propolis, as well as a range of specific flavonoids and flavones, was clearly shown to inhibit the development of a range of viruses including poliovirus and herpes simplex viruses. Flavonols were found to have a greater effect than flavones in the following order of importance: galangin, kaempferol and quercetin. In addition to its effect on virus multiplication, propolis was also found to exert a viricidal action on the enveloped viruses HSV and VSV. The synergy demonstrated by all combinations could explain why propolis is more active than its individual compounds.

In 1992 Serkedjieva,[87] a Bulgarian researcher, tested propolis and some of its fractions on cultures infected with the Hong Kong influenza virus. The greatest effect was achieved when the propolis was applied both before and after infection. In this test phenolic acid derivatives found in propolis also showed activity but no greater than that of whole propolis extract.

CHAPTER 6

Using Propolis to Treat Disease

Testing products *in vitro* can tell us a lot about how products react against particular disease conditions. However, because a product is effective *in vitro* does not always mean that it will be effective *in vivo*, that is in live subjects.

The licensing process for chemical drugs requires strict clinical testing before a drug can go on sale. This involves what are called double blind, placebo-controlled clinical tests on human beings. This means that the new drug has to be clinically tested for its effectiveness on a group of people suffering from the particular disease for which the drug wishes to make a claim to prevent, treat or cure.

At the same time another group of people with the same disease is given a placebo or dummy remedy in order that their response can be compared to that of people taking the drug. Neither group should know whether they are taking the actual drug or the placebo. Everything is done to ensure that the results recorded are real and not imaginary. This exacting, time-consuming and costly process has been designed to assure the public of the safety and efficacy of an essentially synthetic, chemical and, many would argue, intrinsically unnatural form of medicine.

Orthodox medical science argues that nothing less than double blind, placebo-controlled tests can truly verify the value of medicines, natural or otherwise. Few people now believe that this approach is appropriate in exploring the effectiveness of natural medicines like propolis in treating human disease. In what follows we shall draw on a wide range of trials, conducted both in the

East and West, which have explored the wide range of medicinal benefits attributed to propolis.

WHAT USERS THINK ABOUT PROPOLIS

In 1995 a major manufacturer of propolis undertook a survey of people who had purchased propolis products over a six-month period. Whilst this survey of 324 users cannot claim to be a serious scientific study, it does provide some interesting information about what consumers were using propolis for when it first became popular in the UK, and how useful they found it. The study showed the principal uses for propolis were as follows:

- Arthritis and muscular pain 38%
- General health maintenance 24%
- Respiratory problems 18%
- Skin problems 10%
- Chronic fatigue syndrome 6%
- Stomach and digestive disorders 4%

As can be seen, nearly a quarter of users were using propolis for general health maintenance, that is to stay well and, as is illustrated below, to stay free of typical winter ailments—coughs, colds and flu. Of the specific complaints treated with propolis four out of every ten users were taking propolis to help with muscular problems—arthritis and rheumatism—and a further two out of ten for respiratory problems. A further significant number used propolis for treating skin problems like eczema and psoriasis. The figures no doubt reflect the way propolis was publicised in the early days of its popularity but nevertheless confirm the typical use of propolis traditionally.

When asked whether their experience of using the product was positive or negative in treating their particular problem, on average, eight out of ten users said that their experience had been positive. In terms of the specific conditions mentioned above this broke down in the following way.

As well as being the most popular use for propolis, muscular pains was one of the areas where users reported greatest success, with nine of ten reporting a positive response. It also appears that positive results came quickest in this category, with only four out of every

Table 3: Users' experiences with propolis

	POSITIVE	NEGATIVE	TOO SOON
Arthritis and muscular pain	89%	7%	4%
General health maintenance	89%	0%	11%
Respiratory problems	76%	7%	17%
Skin problems	90%	9%	1%
Chronic fatigue syndrome	63%	16%	21%
Stomach and digestive disorders	69%	9%	22%

100 saying it was to soon to say whether the product was helping or not. A similar success pattern was reported when propolis was used for treating skin problems. With less popular uses—chronic fatigue syndrome and digestive disorders—more people (two out of every ten users) reported that it was too soon to tell whether propolis was helping or not despite a significant improvement. As we shall see below, treating these more intractable health problems takes longer and requires a larger intake of propolis.

Propolis users in the survey were asked to comment on how propolis had helped them. Some of these comments are included in full below. They provide a fascinating insight into both the range of uses for propolis and the overwhelmingly positive response to its use.

Arthritis and muscular pain

'Relief from pain, can walk and cycle much better, also walk much further. Only get stiffness in the knee first thing in the morning. Strongly recommend the treatment to other sufferers.'

'Less swelling in joints, feel more comfortable when walking.'

'Relief of pain, also able to walk a lot better. Am able to play more sports and able to cycle.'

'Able to walk better and do not suffer as much pain. Also seem to fight off minor illness more quickly.'

'It has stopped the arthritis getting any worse, it also seems to cure mouth ulcers within a couple of days. It has increased my well-being and the tiredness is a lot less during the day.'

'Since taking the capsules have had relief from pain and generally feel better. Have only been taking the capsules for one month so will definitely carry on.'

'Since taking propolis—has cured chest problems and has definitely helped the arthritis.'

'It has helped to relieve the pain without the sleepy feeling that some tablets have. Used to have injections for the complaint but no longer need them since taking the propolis capsules.'

'Having suffered with arthritis for ten years and suffering a stiff and sore back every morning, since taking propolis this no longer a problem.'

By far the bulk of the responses refer in some way or another to a reduction in the amount of pain and to an increase in mobility, perhaps illustrating the analgesic properties of propolis as well as its anti-inflammatory properties.

Respiratory problems

'Since taking the capsules have had no bad attacks of fighting for breath, still get breathless but not as bad as it was.'

'For two years have not had to resort to painkillers or antibiotics—quite a saving for the NHS.'

'Have had asthma for 16 years, now get over the attacks quicker since taking the capsules which has only been six weeks.'

'Think there is an improvement but it is a bit early to say. Had foot operation two weeks ago and this has healed very quickly.'

'Have been able to reduce steroids intake but have not been able to fully establish the improvement as have only been using propolis for five weeks.'

'They have helped sinus problem but not sure about the asthma. Son has been taking them for ME (Post-viral fatigue syndrome) and they have definitely helped him.'

'After three weeks breathing was much easier so was able to get about much better.'

'Infection cleared up quicker and asthma not as bad.'

'Do not have to use the inhaler as often.'

'Sinuses less blocked, breathing much easier and have not had to use inhaler as much as normal.'

It is interesting to note that as well as helping the specific problem other general health problems have been helped as well.

General health maintenance

'Have only taken the capsules for three weeks, feel 100 per cent better already. Sleeping better and appetite has definitely improved and also helped to relieve breathlessness.'

'Sleeping better, improved skin condition and fewer head colds.'

'Helped to keep colds at bay during the winter.'

'Since taking the capsules have not had a single cold which used to be a regular thing.'

'Have not had any colds for a year now and eczema has totally cleared.'

'After taking propolis for over two years and hardly getting a cold—friend said it was just a coincidence so stopped taking them and suffered the worst winter with numerous colds.'

'Throat and chest have become a lot clearer and feeling better overall. Even hair is getting thicker.'

'Feeling more energetic.'

'Has helped enormously with overall feeling. No longer tired, no throat infections or mouth ulcers which were a regular thing before, nails are stronger and hair is thicker, it even helps with period pains.'

'It has definitely made the immune system stronger, hardly ever get colds now. Treated the dog's eczema with it and it cleared in two–three days.'

'Vast improvement with irritable bowel and slight improvement with nail infection.'

'Have suffered a lot with mouth ulcers, colds, sinus problems, sore throats and cold sores. Since using propolis can honestly say these have been greatly improved, they really help hangover too.'

Skin problems

'Since using the cream there has been a noticeable change within only three days, the skin is less itchy and blotchy.'

'Have suffered with spots and sores for years. Since using the cream there has been a great improvement. Skin is a lot clearer and blemishes have gone. After trying every treatment on the market, propolis is the only cure.'

'Extremely impressed by the effectiveness and speed of the

treatment. Works better than the antibiotics prescribed by the doctor.'

'Completely cured baby's eczema in two applications, also helped daughter's sore knuckles.'

'Have tried all types of creams for psoriasis but never found anything that helped until propolis.'

'The psoriasis is almost clear and the kidneys are showing a slight improvement after renal failure.'

'Rash slowly disappearing and skin much smoother. Better than any prescribed cream.'

'The dermatitis has totally cleared from the hands and 40 per cent improvement to the feet. General health is definitely better from taking the capsules. Skin and hair is greatly improved.'

'Psoriasis has almost cleared up and more energy from taking the capsules.'

'Have been able to stop taking tablets prescribed by the doctors and the acne has improved greatly.'

'Rash cleared completely on one leg and almost gone on the other. Also joint pains have eased off.'

'The scaly patches and unsightly red has totally disappeared.'

'Treating skin condition which the hospital could not help with. Propolis has prevented this spreading and will hopefully clear it completely in time.'

'Facial blemishes have practically gone, have also used the cream for bites and sunburn and it has helped in all cases.'

'Have had rash on face on and off for two years and have tried several creams from the doctor with no success. After using the propolis cream for about a month the rash has cleared, now use the cream nightly and will carry on using.'

Chronic fatigue syndrome

'Getting less infections than usual, less tired and generally feel healthier.'

'It has helped a lot and has definitely built up a resistance to prevent it getting worse.'

'Tiredness has improved greatly and don't get colds and flu as much as usual. Feeling better every day.'

'The fatigue has improved and skin is clearer.'

'Since taking propolis pain in knees has gone, stomach aches are better and feel better overall. Would recommend it to anyone.'

'Less tired and more energy.'

'Look healthier and the aching has got much better. It has also helped the fuzziness that you get with ME. Have had better results than with royal jelly.'

Stomach and digestive disorders

'Practically pain-free and am hopeful that the ulcers have cleared, keeping taking them [capsules] to be absolutely sure.'

'Had serious stomach acid but has now totally cleared.'

'Had just got tablets from the doctor for stomach ulcer when the capsules arrived so took them instead, really looking good and the doctor's tablets are still in the cabinet unopened.'

'Have had great improvement. Digestion has improved and appetite is back.'

'Less pain and not as much heartburn.'

'Cramps related to PMT not so severe and hair seems to have a healthier sheen and generally looks better.'

CLINICAL AND OTHER SCIENTIFIC TRIALS OF PROPOLIS

As this book goes to print, interest in the clinical application of propolis continues to grow, particularly in the West, with interest being increasingly shown from pharmaceutical companies looking for substitutes to chemical drugs. What follows is an alphabetical review of the health problems explored by scientists around the world, but again predominantly in Eastern Europe. In each section the research is referred to in chronological order of publication to provide some idea of the pattern of research in each area. Where known and appropriate, information about how you can treat these problems yourself is provided in each section.

Allergies

Bee products in general have a reputation for triggering allergic reaction. Indeed, one of the very few known side effects of propolis involves just such a reaction. This occurs most often when propolis is used externally, usually in the treatment of skin problems. However, we saw earlier in Dr Bent Havsteen's[1] work how the flavonoids in propolis can also block the allergic response when taken internally. In 1996 Dr Leonard McEwan,[2] a leading allergy specialist in London, reported that patients being treated for allergies using EPD (Enzyme Potentiated Desensitisation), a traditional allopathic treatment, could 'greatly reduce the chance of infection around the time of desensitisation by taking propolis daily for two weeks before EPD, and restarting afterwards and continuing for a further two weeks.' McEwan recommends that patients should start taking propolis not less than seven days before the treatment, and should not restart the treatment until least two weeks after, to avoid sensitising the body to propolis. According to McEwan, propolis causes a temporary alteration in the population of both bacteria and *Candida* in the intestines, increasing their antigens at the start of the treatment.

SELF HELP

Clearly for McEwan propolis has a positive role to play in the treatment of allergies but those who choose to treat themselves must be aware of the possible side effects. (See section, Are there any side effects? in Chapter 7: Propolis Products and their Use.)

Arthritis

The consumer research mentioned earlier showed that propolis was used to treat arthritis more than any other single health problem. Self-medication in this area invariably involves taking propolis internally, either in tincture, capsule or tablet form, or far less frequently via the application of tinctures or creams to the affected areas. Despite this popular use very little research has been conducted in this area.

In 1986 Bulgarian researchers[3] treated 36 patients suffering from various arthritic lesions and traumatic joint disorders. The treatment involved the application of hot wax dressings, enriched with 10 per cent propolis, to the affected areas. Treatment consisted of 10–12 applications each lasting around 30 minutes. In 20 cases, symptoms were decreased by 50–100 per cent, in 14 cases by up to 50 per cent and in two cases were ineffective.

In 1997 researchers, again in Bulgaria[4] treated 42 patients suffering from arthritis, degeneration of joint system with hot compresses of beeswax and propolis. The heat, they claimed, is transmitted to the substratum tissue, improving blood circulation and the metabolic processes in the cartilage and bone tissue. The propolis absorbed by the skin works as an anti-inflammatory and analgesic. The treatment resulted in reduction in swelling around the joint and an increase in joint mobility as well as a reduction in the use of analgesics and non-steroid anti-inflammatory drugs.

SELF HELP

If you cannot find a therapist able to deliver the hot wax and propolis treatment you can either take between 1–2 grams of propolis per day internally or gently massage propolis tincture into the affected area, but note that propolis tincture can stain the skin and clothing.

Asthma

Respiratory problems have traditionally been treated effectively with propolis, and pharmacological research referred to earlier has illustrated the role of propolis in inhibiting the inflammatory process present in respiratory problems.

In 1975 Mihailescu,[5] a Romanian researcher, treated 30 patients suffering from bronchial asthma. Patients were split into two groups, one treated conventionally and the other with propolis. Those treated with propolis showed a marked improvement over those treated conventionally.

Dr Leonard McEwan,[6] the allergy specialist referred to earlier, in particular recommends the use of high doses of propolis to those of his asthma patients who suffer from frequent chest infections, which traditionally require treatment with antibiotics. The propolis should be taken as soon as a cold or infection is suspected. He recommends that the treatment last for at least five days. In the case of chronic sufferers, who often have to be admitted to hospital as emergencies, he recommends continuous treatment with propolis. Clinical rcsearch is currently in progress in the Asthma Unit at Barnsley General Hospital in the UK.

SELF HELP
Dr McEwan advises approximately 1.5 grams per daily use. This can be take either as a capsule or in tablet form. Some asthma suffers report that propolis tincture can have a more immediate effect when sufferers believe an asthmatic attack to be imminent.

Bedsores

In 1978 Serbanescu,[7] a Romanian doctor used a 10 per cent propolis powder in 80 per cent inert powder for treating a group of 12 patients with severe multiple sacral bedsores. This treatment was compared with the conventional treatment of a further 12 patients. In the group treated with propolis nine out of 12 showed very good results with chronic bedsores being cured in 16–54 days. In the three cases which did not clear up, they at least did not get worse. In the control group only three patients were cured and in a longer period (43–75 days). The same doctors also used a propolis spray with 5–10 and 20 per cent propolis concentrations to treat patients before the eruption of bedsores, with considerable success. Following cessation of the treatment, bedsores re-appeared.

In 1999, Stojko[8,9] at the University of Silesia treated 96 cases of bedsores with propolis. Patients were treated twice a day using a three per cent propolis and wax balm. The treatment was noted as being more effective than traditional treatments as observed in the more rapid granulation of tissue and the healing-over of the ulcerous tissue. No allergic responses were noted.

SELF HELP

A few propolis sprays are on the market. You can also find out how to make your own in Chapter 10: Making Your Own Medicines. Good quality propolis creams may also be helpful, particularly when used as a preventative.

Bone regeneration

Propolis has traditionally been used to help bone knit together In 1978, Polish doctors[10] tested this theory on animals. An ethanolic extract of propolis was injected into the radial leg bones of some dogs. They claim that the regeneration of the bone tissue was about twice as fast as in the untreated controls.

In 1985, again in Poland,[10] similar research was conducted but this time with human subjects. Twenty-two patient with Legg-Calve-Perthes disease (of the hip joint) were injected with an aqueous extract of propolis. Thirty-two other patients were given a conventional treatment. The patients treated with propolis showed significantly greater improvement than the control group. Whilst no research has as yet been undertaken, it would be interesting to look at the role of propolis in treating osteoporosis (brittle bone disease) including its common association with the menopause.

SELF HELP

Regular intake of propolis throughout the day, up to a maximum of 3 grams, for two–three weeks following breaking of bone.

Bronchitis

We have seen that, traditionally, honeycomb cappings, which contain quantities of propolis, have been used for treating bronchitis.

In 1975 Russian doctors[11] reported on their treatment of 76 children with non-specific pneumonia between 1964–1969. This research is especially interesting because it compared the effectiveness of antibiotics alone, with antibiotics combined with propolis. The propolis treatment was administered using an aerosol. The best results were found in the group using a combination of antibiotics and a 100 per cent water-based propolis solution.

In 1989 Dr Scheller[12] at the Silesian Medical School treated 260 steelworkers suffering from bronchitis. Patients were treated for 24 days, some with conventional methods and others with an ethanol extract of propolis (EEP) in a physiological salt solution. The best results were obtained in patients treated with the propolis liquid together with propolis tablets.

Again in 1989 Russian researchers[13] treated 104 patients with chronic bronchitis. Conventional methods were used in the treatment of 56 patients while 48 patients received honey-and-propolis inhalations in addition to conventional therapy. The patients receiving the propolis-and-honey treatment were discharged three–four days earlier than those treated conventionally. The rate of relapse amongst the conventionally-treated patients was also twice that of those treated with propolis.

SELF HELP

Honey, too, has a range of anti-bacterial properties. Combining the two as shown above can be effective as well as making the propolis more palatable. For general use, see Asthma.

Burns

The use of honey in the treatment of burns has been common amongst natural practitioners for centuries. It is possible its perceived potency was related to the presence of propolis when raw and untreated honey was used.

The first recorded medical use of propolis in treating burns was in 1962 at the Rachfuss Children's Hospital, Leningrad, USSR.[14] Dr Zabeklina recommended its use in treating infected wounds in children.

In 1975 doctors[15] at the Russian Central Hospital for the Treatment of Burns and Scalds reported on the treatment of burns patients with propolis over a ten-year period. The ointment was prepared using 15 per cent propolis with any fat or oil (animal or vegetable) but was most frequently made with a combination of peach, apricot and sunflower oils. The hospital treated 830 patients between 1961 and 1970. They found that the ointments had anaesthetic, bactericidal and regenerative effects on wounds as well as limiting the surface area of the scars. They also improved blood circulation and lymphatic circulation. They found that the propolis dressings did not stick to the wound and did not provoke trauma on the granulations.

In 1986 Grochowski[16], a Polish doctor, used a three per cent propolis ointment containing soya oil, dehydrated butter and beeswax on mice suffering from skin burns. He found that burns treated with the propolis ointment healed much quicker than the ones treated conventionally.

The most recent research was reported in 1997 by Cuban researchers[17] at the 35th International Apicultural Congress in Antwerp. In 1993 because of a severe shortage of burns drugs nationally in Cuba, the health service approached the Experimental Apicultural Institute in Cuba, for help in developing an appropriate bee product. Burn treatment with alcohol extract of propolis is not recommended because of the secondary burns created by the alcohol so the researchers looked for an alternative. The station developed a honey-and-propolis mixture which has proved significantly more effective than using propolis alone.

SELF HELP

Minor burns can be treated with a variety of propolis creams, ointments, tinctures or sprays. If a tincture is used it is best not to use an alcohol-based one but rather one with a propylene glycol base.

Colitis

In 1975 Bulgarian researchers[18] used EEP to treat 45 patients with acute and chronic colitis. The results were very good for 26 patients, good for 12 and satisfactory in five cases. Only for two patients was there no beneficial result. Pain diminished in most cases by the seventh day of treatment, disappearing completely by the 19–20th day. In all cases the sensation of pressure in the abdomen disappeared after the fifth day of treatment.

SELF HELP

It is not known how the EEP was delivered but the most likely way would be orally. Take the tincture in warm liquid on an empty stomach.

Coughs and colds

As the consumer research quoted earlier shows, a high proportion of users take propolis on a regular basis to stay well, to maintain a strong immune system and ward off coughs, colds and flu. Ironically, very little clinical work appears to have been done in this area. In 1989 Polish researchers[19] looked at the effects of propolis on the common cold. The group treated with propolis had the infection for a shorter period, with complete recovery within three days. The untreated group required five days to recover.

SELF HELP

Best results seem to be obtained by taking between 1–1.5 grams of propolis per day, every day. Some authorities suggest that people taking propolis continually should take a break of a week or so every three or four months to prevent the body become oversensitized to it.

Dental problems

Propolis has been a traditional treatment for dental problems for hundreds of years. Perhaps because of this, and also because the effect of treatment is relatively easy to identify, it has also become one of the most popular areas of clinical research into the use of propolis in both East and West.

In 1980 Dr Schmidt,[20] a German researcher, conducted a double-blind clinical trial of a propolis mouthwash. The study showed those patients with gingivitis (inflammation of the gums) and periodontal disease showed significant improvement after four weeks' use, assessed by the level of plaque formation and gum inflammation. The mouthwash consisted of one part of 1:10 propolis liquid in five parts of water, taken morning and evening. Romanian researchers[21] in 1983 produced a propolis-and-royal jelly product (Gingiprop) which they used successfully to treat gingivitis. A similar product based on propolis (Propolan) was developed by Cuban researchers[22] in 1986 and was used successfully in the treatment of chronic gingivitis. German researchers[23] in the same year, in a study of the development of plaque and gingivitis, found that propolis can be a useful adjunct to oral hygiene.

A study carried out on dogs in 1987 in Yugoslavia[24] showed that propolis increased the flow of blood to dental pulp. Further experimental work on the teeth of calves in 1988 in Czechoslovakia[25] illustrated that propolis both reduced inflammation and stimulated the healing process.

In 1989 Dr Gafar[26] from Romania, used propolis to treat chronic oral cavity problems comparing its effect with other natural products used in dental hygiene. He found that propolis was effective in treating inflammation of the gums and oral mucous membrane as well as helping scars to heal effectively. A Russian study in 1990[27] recommended the use of propolis in root canal fillings because of its anaesthetic and bone-regenerating properties. In the same year a Romanian study[28] showed that a paste consisting of propolis and zinc oxide, used to cap dental pulp, increased the production of dentin and encouraged the remineralisation of the bone.

Another study using animals, carried out at a Japanese university in 1991,[29] found that rats given propolis in water showed significantly less dental caries than rats not treated with the propolis.

The use of propolis in mainstream dentistry in the UK has grown considerably over the last few years, mainly as a result of the work of Philip Wander,[30] who runs a number of dental practices in Manchester. He has been a constant champion of the use of propolis for a wide range of problems. In a study published in 1995 he reports the experiences of a growing number of his colleagues in the UK, who are using propolis to treat oral ulceration (50 cases), denture trauma, herpetic and non-specific painful oral ulcerations. The treatment involves the application of a strong (50 per cent) propolis tincture direct to the infected areas. The treatment can be taken over by the patient. He found that ulcers healed within two days. Periodontal inflammation caused by erupting wisdom teeth was also treated. Propolis is recommended as a mouthwash and breath freshener. He also recommends the use of propolis as an antiseptic handscrub for dental surgery.

Similarly encouraging results were reported in 1996 by dentist Peter Varley[31] in a postgraduate research paper.

SELF HELP

Propolis tincture is used either as a mouthwash or gargle or applied directly to the infected areas. Raw propolis, providing it is clean and of good quality, can be chewed and when plastic, formed round the painful tooth.

Diabetes

In 1997 a team of Chinese researchers led by Fu-hai Liu[32] published research into the use of a complex blend of bee products, designed to treat diabetes. They describe what they refer to as *Fengzhen*, 'a new type of complex medicine prepared from bee pollen and propolis.' They claim that it can help to control the level of blood sugars and blood fats. They also claim that Fengzhen can soften blood vessels and improve blood circulation as well as preventing and curing the complications of diabetes.

The same team of researchers[33] treated 57 patients suffering from diabetes mellitus with propolis alone. Patients included 50 with NIDDM (non-insulin dependent diabetes mellitus) and seven with IDDM (insulin-dependent diabetes mellitus). The group was randomly divided into three, with one group receiving traditional pharmaceutical treatment and the others receiving the propolis treatment. After three months' observation researchers observed that the reduction in blood sugar levels among those receiving the propolis treatment was no worse than among those receiving the classical treatment, but that the process was quicker with propolis. They also observed that the propolis treatment had a beneficial effect on diabetes patients with periodontitis and oral cavity fungal infections.

Eyes

In 1978 Romanian researchers[34] reported on the use of a two–five per cent propolis ophthalmic solution and an ointment containing 5–10 per cent of propolis to treat various eye problems. They claim these products produced excellent results in treating burns and injuries to the eye when applied to surrounding tissues. Both products were effective against microbial and viral inflammatory infections of the eyes. They replaced distilled water with a 10 per cent solution of Macrodex, which they suggest caused less irritation to the eye.

In 1997 the Romanian, Popescu,[35] reviewed 21 years' of treatment of eye problems involving over 100,000 patients at the Ophthalmic Apitherapy Department of the Bee Research Institute in Bucharest. During this period Popescu developed a range of eyewashes based on bee products, including honey, royal jelly and propolis. The eyewashes were tested on animals before use in the clinic. The conditions that responded best included conjunctivitis, blepharitis, keratopathy, and corneal ulcers of a viral origin, iridocyclitis and cataracts in the first and second evolution stages. The authors suggest that treatment with bee products was effective in over 85 per cent of the cases.

Flu

Flu is a viral infection which is notoriously difficult to treat once contracted. Consumers report that they are less likely to catch flu if they are taking propolis and if they do get it they suffer less. In 1954, Dr Iojris, author of *Healing Properties of Honey and Bee Pollen*[36] told us that this viral infection of the respiratory tract can cause fever, headache and weakness, and can be dangerous when complicated by bacterial infection of the lungs. Treatment with propolis extract, he claimed, was found to provide prophylactic protection against the virus.

The prophylactic effect of propolis would seem to be confirmed by the Russian Shevchenko's[37] research in 1972. In this research he found that feeding mice with propolis prior to exposure to influenza protected them against the infection but was not as effective once they had got it. Similar research in Romania[38] and Bulgaria[39] confirmed the prophylactic effect of propolis treatment on mice when subsequently exposed to the virus.

Perhaps the most dramatic test of the effectiveness of propolis against influenza took place during an epidemic of influenza in Sarajevo, Yugoslavia, in 1978. During the epidemic Professor Osmanagic[40] conducted a trial amongst students at a nursing college, who had been exposed to patients with flu. Eighty students took propolis while 182 did not. Of those who took propolis, only seven per cent became ill whilst 63 per cent of those who did not take the propolis contracted influenza. Similar success was reported in another study, also in Yugoslavia, in 1978[41].

SELF HELP

Take 1.5 grams daily in tablet or capsule form to stay well. Increase the dose when ill. Fifteen drops of tincture can also be taken three times a day in warm water or in juice.

Fungal Infections

In 1978 Chinese researchers at the Workers Hospital, Kangsu, China[42] tested a 1–10 per cent alcohol extract of propolis against a range of fungal infections. The propolis treatment was found to be effective against ten superficial fungi but not against *Trichophyton* and nine deep-growing fungi. Russian researchers[43] in 1979 treated 12 patients with chronic fungal sinusitis caused by *Candida albicans* with an alcohol oil emulsion of propolis. After five–eight treatments clinical recovery occurred in nine cases and improvement in three. Recovery occurred after 10–17 days.

SELF HELP

Use creams or tincture if you do not mind the skin being stained. Rub gently into the affected area. Check with patch test for allergy first.

Gastrointestinal disorders

Dr Makarov,[44] the Russian author of *Propolis Therapy* used propolis to treat nausea, heartburn, poor appetite, hyperacidity (too much acid) and hypoacidity (too little acid). Patients were given 20 drops of propolis tincture three times a day. After five days all patients were relieved of pain and acidity became normalised. Dr Makarov recommended propolis for the treatment of ulcers (abscesses) in the stomach and/or duodenum. 'Recovery', he claims, 'occurs more quickly with treatment by propolis than it does with the use of common medicines.'

In 1997 Russian researchers[45] reported on their treatment with propolis of 48 children between the ages of two and a half months and three years, with lingering intestinal infections. Typically, this inflammatory condition involves the destruction of enterocytes, the modification of normal intestinal flora and the breakdown of general and local immunity. A 10 per cent solution of propolis was used to treat the children. Thirty-five of the children (75 per cent) improved markedly. Intoxication symptoms disappeared, the frequency of stools decreased and the children put on weight. In the group not treated with propolis only 40 per cent showed good clinical response.

SELF HELP

Weak propolis tincture taken in warm water taken at regular intervals throughout the day.

Hangovers

In 1990 a patent was issued in Japan[46] for a product containing propolis, which claimed to cure hangovers as well as the symptoms of asthma and allergies. No research data is available to support this claim.

Hay fever

Consumer research indicates that a number of users found relief from hay fever when taking propolis. In 1980 Dr Remy Chauvin,[47] the French physician noted for his championing of propolis, treated a number of patients with hay fever. The patients were treated with an alcohol extract of propolis in soluble starch. Each patient received seven–eight doses daily for eight days, each dose containing 250mgs of dry propolis extract. The patients' symptoms were almost completely alleviated. Small doses were given in the following two years with continuing positive results.

SELF HELP
As above or take an equal amount in capsule, tablet or tincture form. Discontinue if the unpleasant symptoms of allergic reaction are experienced.

Hearing

Using propolis to treat hearing problems is one of its more unusual applications. Russian doctors[48] in 1973 treated 382 patients with various ear diseases and defects using a 30–40 per cent tincture of propolis mixed with olive oil or maize oil in a ratio of 1:4. Gauze earplugs soaked in the creamy solution were left for three days in the patients' ears. The treatment was repeated 10–12 times. Three hundred and fourteen patients showed improved hearing and fewer patients reported head noises after treatment.

In 1975 Popnikolov[49] in Bulgaria, treated 40 patients with suppurative swelling of the inner ear. Hearing had been affected in most cases. An extract of 30g of propolis in 100g of alcohol was applied to the infected areas. In 80 per cent of the cases suppuration stopped, the smell decreased and hearing became sharper.

Between 1968 and 1973 Russian doctors[50] treated 68 patients with acute inflammation of the inner ear using an alcohol extract of propolis. The treatment was successful in 94 per cent of the cases.

SELF HELP

Clearly, caution must be exercised when placing anything in the ear. Cotton wool can be used instead of gauze.

Herpes

Herpes is a viral disease, which manifests itself often as painful blisters on the site of nerve tracts. It is commonly known as shingles. Dr Franz Feiks,[51] an Austrian doctor, used a five per cent solution of EEP applied with a brush to treat 21 cases. In all of the 21 cases treated, pain disappeared within 48 hours and itching persisted for only three days following the treatment. Application of a propolis spray did not work as effectively.

In 1988 Dr Giurcaneanu[52] of the Dermatological Service Bucharest, Romania, found that the application of propolis products had a significant effect against recurrent herpes and zona zoster. Improvement was noted as reduced duration of the lesions, reduced pain and increased interval between recurrence of lesions.

In a Canadian trial in 1995 at Winnipeg General Hospital[53] 50 patients were treated for herpes labialis (mouth), half of them with a placebo and half receiving a patented propolis cream product, ACF, developed in Poland. The average recovery days in the propolis-treated group was 3.84 days whilst in the control it was 8.52.

SELF HELP

Propolis tincture or cream can be applied externally as in the tests above. Remember that propolis tincture can stain both skin and clothing. Propolis may be taken internally at the same time.

Hypertension/heart

In 1978 45 patients were treated with propolis at the Workers Hospital, Kiangsu Province, China.[54] Conditions treated included high blood pressure, arteriosclerosis and coronary heart disease. 'Promising results' were claimed but some side effects were noted.

In experiments using animals at a medical school in Poland in 1999,[55] rats were fed a preparation of honey, propolis and pollen in order to test whether this would reduce artificially induced high levels of fat in their diet. The treatment resulted in statistically significant reductions in the blood fat levels in the rats.

Immune support/ME

German research in 1988,[56] identified the way in which the bio-flavonoids in propolis stimulate the production of interferon, which is important in the maintenance of a strong immune system.

In 1996 Dr Leonard McEwan[57] reported on his treatment of 27 patients suffering from ME (Post-viral fatigue syndrome) with high doses of propolis. Within four months of commencing treatment 24 patients had 'obtained a major benefit', 14 patients were able to return to work, college, school, etc. and resume physical activity which had previously been impossible. Of this 14, six relapsed within eight weeks of stopping the propolis treatment or of reducing intake to 500mg or less per day. McEwan emphasises the importance of continuing high doses—a minimum of 1.5 grams per day—if the treatment is to be successful. He advises that treatment should continue for at least one year.

In 1997 the UK National ME (Myalgic Encephalomyelitis) Association[58] published the results of a survey on the use of propolis by their members. Fifty-eight people with ME, aged between 26 and 67, took part in the survey. All were diagnosed as having had ME for between 11 months and 14 years. Of the 58 participants in the survey, 12 said they were severely ill (bed-bound or housebound) while 20 were very ill. Of the remainder, four were only mildly affected and six felt they were on the road to recovery. They took between 1–12 grams of propolis per day in capsules, tablets and tinctures. Fifty-three reported that taking propolis had made a difference to their ME, usually immediately, but certainly within the first two weeks. Four people reported no difference and one reported an adverse reaction.

Of 22 people who reported reducing or stopping propolis treatment, 18 reported deterioration followed by an improvement once they restarted the treatment. Those taking 1000mg or less reported least benefit. The authors suggest that the most effective amount was around 3000mg per day, although more severely affected patients only reported benefits from taking between 8–12g per day. Patients reported increase in energy, greater mobility and a reduction in infections.

Between 1994 and 1997, ACOBOS[59] a counselling organisation in Nairobi (part of the Kenyan National Aids Control Programme), began supplying propolis capsules along with counselling to people suffering from HIV and full blown AIDS. In a short report the author details the general improvement in health and appetite amongst sufferers which in some cases led to the resumption of a normal life and a return to work.

SELF HELP

A minimum of 3g of good quality propolis is required per day. (See ME Association findings.) This can be taken in tablet, capsule or tincture form.

Low back pain

Low back pain is one of the most common ailments for which people seek over-the-counter treatment in the UK.

Bulgarian researchers[60] in 1997 reported on their treatment of 22 patients between the ages of 32–60, all with low back pain. Beeswax and propolis were mixed in a ratio of one part propolis to ten parts wax. Gauze compresses were soaked in the melted mixture and applied to the affected area whilst still hot. The compresses were left in place for between 25–30 minutes. The procedure was repeated between 12 and 15 times. Eight patients had considerable improvement and 14 experienced improvement according to various objective tests. Similar research in 1991,[61] also in Bulgaria, reported equally positive results from this treatment.

Parasites

In 1988 Cuban researchers[62] successfully treated 138 patients with a propolis extract (Propolisina) for giardiasis (a protozoal infection). No side effects were observed.

Pharyngitis/laryngitis and sore throats

In 1971 Russian scientists[63] used a 15 per cent extract of propolis to treat 260 cases of pharyngitis. Sixty-seven per cent were completely cured, 28 per cent showed some improvement and only four per cent showed no improvement.

In 1975, Doroshenko,[64] at Clinical Hospital No. 11, Kiev, USSR, treated 238 pharyngitis patients with a propolis mixture. One part of 30 per cent extract of propolis was mixed with glycerine (or peach oil) and applied to the mucous membrane of the infected area over a period of 10–15 days. Seventy-five per cent made a complete recovery while 14 per cent substantially. The researchers found that the propolis extract enhanced the effect of most pharmaceutical drugs used in the treatment of pharyngitis.

Romanian researchers[65] in the same year used propolis in the treatment of 200+ patients with acute pharyngitis, acute tonsillitis and acute laryngitis. In each treatment group 10 per cent of the patients were treated by normal methods. Patients treated with propolis recovered more quickly than the control group.

Again in Romania, in 1975 Matel[66] and others treated a variety of mucous membrane inflammations including ulcers and labial herpes. Thirty-four patients received treatment with propolis liquid and propolis tablets. The propolis liquid was found to have anti-viral, anaesthetic, anti-bacterial and mycotic effects.

SELF HELP

Traditionally, the treatment of sore throats has been a favourite use for propolis. Treatment can be by a variety of forms. Gargle with a solution of propolis tincture and warm water and swallow the solution for added effect, coating the throat with propolis. A range of commercially produced propolis throat lozenges are also available but these often have only a small percentage of propolis and at best used to treat only mild inflammations.

Prostate inflammation

Increasing interest has been shown in recent years in the use of a range of bee products—propolis, pollen and royal jelly—to treat prostate problems.

In 1997 Mladenov[67] and colleagues in Bulgaria treated 55 patients aged between 55 and 95 all suffering from prostate hypertrophy. All of them had been recommended for surgery under conventional treatment. The authors designed individual treatment programmes using a combination of honey, pollen, propolis and royal jelly. After one or two months treatment 95 per cent of the patients no longer complained of pain and their prostates had returned to normal size. One 93-year-old who had had a catheter introduced six months prior to treatment recovered sufficiently for the catheter to be removed.

Finally, in 1999, a Russian researcher, Saraf[68] reported on his treatment of 36 patients with acute and chronic prostatitis. Again the treatment involved a combination of propolis, royal jelly, beebread and honey delivered via by suppositories. Eighty-nine per cent of this treatment group improved significantly, with reduced pain and improved function according to scientifically-approved basic blood and urine tests.

Radiation

Doctors at the Institute of Radiology, Sarajevo, Yugoslavia,[69] used propolis to treat a number of patients with serious liver damage caused by irradiation complications, including the over-use of X-rays. They found that the radiation problems lessened or disappeared in this double-blind placebo-controlled test.

Skin problems—psorasis, eczema, acne, etc.

Two out of ten people in the consumer survey referred to earlier used propolis to successfully treat a variety of skin problems, relying no doubt on its anti-inflammatory properties as described in the pharmacology section.

In 1962, Dr Zabelina[70] at the Rachfuss Children's Hospital,

Leningrad, USSR, treated children with infected wounds or newborn children with tissue disorders using a propolis salve. Dr Zabelina reported that the treatment was able to curb inflammation and disinfect wounds as well as stimulate new growth.

Danilov,[71] a Russian doctor, in 1975 reported his use of propolis in treating 680 patients with skin problems. Problems included eczema, neurodermatitis and ulcers. In 90 per cent of the cases the treatment using a propolis ointment was successful. Again in Russia, Drs Vinogradova and Zajceva[72] found propolis useful in treating a range of minor skin problems: 'Bee propolis preparations worked particularly well with patients who had limited chronic neurodermatitis characterised by frequent recurrence.'

Dr Edith Lauda,[73] an Austrian, used propolis tincture and ointment to treat acne and other dermatological problems. One woman with acne pustolus affecting her whole face, which had not responded to chemotherapy, was completely cured within two weeks following treatment. In 1996, Dr McEwan[74] used a weak propolis solution (around two per cent propolis in solution) to successful treat acne and local skin infections.

Finally, in 1999 researchers at the Dermatological Institute, Nizhny Novgorod, Russia,[75] treated a variety of chronic skin problems including neurodermatitis and chronic eczema with a propolis-and-royal jelly cream. The cream was applied twice a day. The skin became less dry and began to grow, peeling off the skin was reduced, and erithema and other features of inflammation diminished after five–seven days of application. No allergic responses were noted.

SELF HELP

A large range of propolis products are available to treat a variety of skin problems like eczema, psoriasis, etc. Propolis creams can be applied externally (always try the patch test first to see you are allergic). You can also take propolis internally to boost your general health and assist the healing process.

Smallpox

In 1975 Krivoruchko,[76] a Russian doctor found that propolis was very effective in *in vitro* tests against smallpox vaccine. Limited effectiveness was found in human patients but only when the propolis was taken before the infection.

Tuberculosis

In 1975 Russian doctors[77] reported on their treatment of 147 cases of broncho-pulmonary tuberculosis, including tubercular adenopathy, trachea bronchitis, kidney tuberculosis, and other forms of tuberculoderm. One hundred and seven cases were treated solely with propolis administered in a variety of forms. Propolis was found to be 'an efficient additional substance in the complex treatment of tuberculosis.'

By the late 1980s tuberculosis was thought to have finally been brought under control. It has, however, emerged again in recent years in the UK and in other Western countries, in strains difficult if not impossible to treat with conventional drugs. It may be that propolis taken alongside conventional medicines can help.

Trephination

This is perhaps the most unusual medical use of propolis. Trephination involves the drilling of small holes in the skull to relieve pressure and for a variety of other reasons. Doctors at the Kiev Medical Institute, USSR,[78] used a 10 per cent alcohol solution of propolis or a 33 per cent propolis ointment to reduce infection around the trephination cavities. They found that propolis was highly effective against gram-negative bacteria on trephination cavities. Favourable results were obtained in 89 per cent of cases while 11 per cent showed no improvement.

Ulcers

The relatively recent discovery that stomach ulcers may be caused by bacteria has led to a number of alternative treatments being put forward. Research in New Zealand showed that Manuka honey was particularly effective. Dr Franz Feiks[79] was one of the first to treat stomach ulcers with propolis. Patients were given a five per cent extract of propolis three times a day. The group taking propolis showed a decrease in pain after three days. After ten days six out of ten patients showed no evidence of wounds in the stomach.

In 1983 Korsun,[80] a Russian researcher, treated 64 patients aged between 23 and 98 years with tibial skin ulcers. The treatment involved the application of a mixture of propolis tincture and calendula tincture, homogenized and mixed with vaseline. The ointment was applied daily to the ulcerated area. The periphery of the ulcer was also treated with antibiotic ointments. The treatment lasted 12 weeks. At the end of the treatment, 19 patients showed no signs of the condition, 19 showed an improved condition and in nine there was no change or a worsening of their condition.

Peptic ulcers were again successfully treated with propolis by Gorbatenko[81] in 1971. The propolis treatment effectively reduced inflammation of the upper gastrointestinal tract.

Romanian researchers[82] in 1978 reported on their treatment of 34 patients with chronic external ulcers. A variety of propolis preparations were used, including ointments and propolis in oil and glycerine. Fifteen cases were completely cured, 13 cases showed satisfactory progress and in six cases the treatment was stopped because of the development of eczema.

SELF HELP

Propolis cream or propolis tincture (a non-alcoholic tincture will sting less) can be applied round the outside of the ulcer on a daily basis. Do the patch test first, however, to establish whether you are allergic.

Urinary tract infection

This increasingly common condition, especially in women, is treated conventionally with repeated doses of antibiotics. Dr L. McEwan[83] found that continuous treatment with propolis may give adequate protection to sufferers with persistent cases of urinary tract infection as well as to women who suffer from repeated infections of the bladder and kidneys. Dr McEwan claims this treatment is often preferable to the long-term use of antibiotics.

SELF HELP

Propolis can be taken internally in any form—liquid, capsule or tablet. Dr McEwan recommends a minimum of 1.5g per day.

Women's problems

In the 1995 consumer survey a number of women reported that pre-menstrual tension and cramps had improved after taking propolis and it may be that this is an area where further research would be valuable. However, the majority of research in this area relates to the treatment of infections and inflammatory conditions of the female genitalia.

In 1971, doctors at the Department of Obstetrics, Kiev Hospital, in the USSR,[84] used propolis successfully for treating wounds in women following childbirth. Again in Russia[85] women suffering from erosion of the neck of the uterus, irritated cervix and other vaginal problems were treated with a propolis solution. Propolis was found to be 98 per cent successful after 12 days of treatment.

Polish researchers[86] reported in 1973 that propolis was effective against purulent vaginal inflammation.

Dr Suchy[87] of the Department of Obstetrics, Zdroy, Poland, reports the disappearance of symptoms in cases of uterine neck inflammation caused by the parasite *Trichomonas vaginalis* following local application of 30mg propolis vaginal tablets. Suchy also records the successful treatment of female students with dysmenorrhea (painful menstruation) in 50 out of 60 cases treated. The propolis salve used had no toxic properties or irritant reaction and quickly and effectively stimulated the epithelialisation of the affected areas.

In 1989, Roman and others[88] described the treatment of 57 patients between the ages of 21 and 58 with ulcero-erosive cervicitis, sometimes accompanied by *Candida* infections and other inflammatory conditions. Patients were treated with local applications of propolis ointments, tincture sprays and ovules. Excellent results were obtained with 42 patients (76.3 per cent), satisfactory results with nine (16.4 per cent) and no result with three. Three patients were excluded because of allergic response.

In 1997 Bulgarian researchers[89] reported on treatment given to 60 women between the ages of 40 and 60 with cervical arthrosis. They were all treated using an ointment containing an alcohol solution of 30 per cent propolis with lanolin and Vaseline. During the treatment subjective improvements were observed, including a perceived reduction in pain. Following treatment the clinical condition of 32 patients returned completely to normal and improved with 28 subjects

Also from Bulgaria, Panova and others[90] reported on their treatment of 524 women with a variety of gynaecological diseases, principally pre-cancerous erosions of the uterus and cervix. The women were treated with a three per cent solution of propolis in 96 per cent alcohol. The results were good in both women under and over the age of 40. The authors concluded: 'propolis has a well established place in the treatment of gynaecological infections.'

SELF HELP

Propolis salve and tincture can be used externally for treatment of wounds and capsules, tablets and tinctures for internal use.

Wounds

We have seen how propolis gained an early reputation for treating wounds during Napoleon's campaign against Russia, during the Boer War, and later during the Second World War followed by the pioneering research at the Kazan Veterinary Institute in the early 1950s.

Scheller,[91] the Polish researcher, reported in 1980 that the topical use of propolis on surgical wounds, burns and ulcers achieved up to 80 per cent faster healing when compared with conventional treatments.

Damyanliev[92] conducted trials in the early 1980s on hospitalized patients with infected wounds. He showed that external treatment with propolis accelerated wound healing and that infection of the wounds was greatly reduced with nearly half of the infecting microbes disappearing after four days. Russian research[93] in 1985 confirmed that patients with infected wounds improved with the external use of propolis together with routine treatment.

Further research by Scheller in 1985[94] showed that when propolis was injected into the necrotic hip joints of patients with Legg-Calve-Perthe disease it greatly assisted healing in conjunction with conventional treatment.

SELF HELP

Apply non-alcohol propolis tincture or strong propolis creams daily around the outside of the wound.

CHAPTER 7

Propolis Products and their Use

MEDICINAL PRODUCTS

As awareness of propolis has grown and commercial companies have entered the market, so the range of products has increased to the point where you can now buy propolis in a huge variety of forms. This has made the use of propolis far easier. However, the commercial product with all its packaging and hype can create an unnecessary mystique. The basis of most of these products is very simple and you can made them yourself if you are inclined. (See Chapter 10: Making Your Own Medicines.) All the commercial products listed below have traditionally been obtainable through health stores and are increasingly available through pharmacies.

PROPOLIS CAPSULES (HARD GEL)

Powdered propolis, often mixed with pollen or some other filler, is encapsulated in two-piece hard gelatine, or increasingly vegetable matter, capsules.
Use: Taken internally to treat a variety of health problems.

PROPOLIS CAPSULES (SOFT GEL)

These are one-piece gelatine capsules, filled with a propolis liquid, often mixed with some other compound such as soya oil or paste.
Use: Taken internally to treat a variety of health problems.

PROPOLIS LIQUIDS

The basic liquids used are alcohol, propylene glycol and water. (See section in chapter 9 on Extracting and Refining Propolis.) In some cases other products may be added to either give greater value to the product, e.g. other bee products (royal jelly, honey, bee bread) or herbal mixtures (echinacea, ginseng, etc.) or to alter the taste, e.g. lemon juice or liquorice or honey.

Use: The liquids can be used both internally and externally. Used internally, they are thought to have a greater bio-availability, i.e. because the propolis is already a liquid, it enters the body more quickly. You can also use the liquid as part of a gargle for treating sore throats or dental problems.

The pure liquids may also be used externally for treating wounds, burns and skin problems. However, care must be taken when using an alcoholic liquid on open wounds as the alcohol stings. In such cases use either a non-alcoholic product or gently dab the product round the outside of the affected area first. When used externally, it is advisable to first test the product on a patch of skin to check that you are not allergic. It should be noted that propolis liquid does leave a brown stain on the skin and any clothing it comes into contact with.

PROPOLIS SYRUPS

These are usually made from propolis mixed with a variety of sweet carriers—honey, glycerine, maple syrup, etc.

Use: Syrups are mostly used for treatment of coughs and are a particularly effective way of delivering propolis to children.

PROPOLIS LOZENGES

In most cases these are candy or sweets containing small quantities of propolis, along with sugar, honey, artificial sweeteners and sometimes natural or artificial flavourings.

Use: For alleviation of sore throats. They are, however, not the most effective way of treating these conditions. They may also be effective in treating halitosis (bad breath).

PROPOLIS CHEWING GUM

One American company has patented a propolis chewing gum which it claims aids dental hygiene. One UK company has even branded their product Dental Gum.

Use: Whether these products add a great deal to dental hygiene given the sweeteners they contain is not known. Using propolis as a mouthwash or gargle is likely to be more effective if less convenient.

PROPOLIS ORAL AND NASAL SPRAYS AND AEROSOLS

These products are essentially propolis liquids in a solution (usually alcohol) thin enough to allow them to be delivered through a spray or aerosol.

Use: Internally, they are used to treat sore throats, inflamed nasal passages, as a breath freshener and for treating dental problems. They are especially useful in treating mouth ulcers. Externally, they can be used to apply propolis to fungal infections.

PROPOLIS CREAMS

A large number of propolis creams are available on the market today. These are normally natural cream bases with one–two per cent propolis liquid added.

Use: These creams are mainly used to treat dermatological problems like psoriasis and eczema, but can also be used as a gentle antiseptic cream to treat wounds and burns where the skin has not broken. Some people use propolis cream as an anti-ageing cream believing that it helps to retain the elasticity of skin collagen.

PROPOLIS OINTMENTS

These are normally made from refined propolis mixed with a range of vegetable or animal fats or oils.

Use: Normally used for the external treatment of skin problems, wounds, burns, etc.

PROPOLIS TOOTHPASTE

Several companies now produce a propolis toothpaste, made by mixing small quantities of propolis—around one per cent—with traditional toothpaste bases. Propolis toothpastes are also

frequently mixed with other flavourings or healing herbs or resins—frankincense, peppermint and myrrh—either for their medicinal properties or as a flavouring.
Use: For routine dental hygiene.

PROPOLIS SHAMPOO

Propolis has been added to basic shampoo mixtures and marketed in the same way as other herbal shampoos, as an invigorating, nourishing and sometimes antiseptic treatment for the scalp and hair. Consumer research has shown that taking propolis internally has led to better quality hair.
Use: Used as with a normal shampoo. Not many of these products are on the market, perhaps because too much propolis can stain the hair.

PROPOLIS SOAP

Many natural soaps containing propolis have been produced by blending propolis, usually with natural soap recipes, either as a hard soap or as liquid soap.
Use: Normally used in the same way as other 'medicated' soaps. They are suitable for maintaining a healthy skin and for the treatment of acne.

SOME COMMONLY ASKED QUESTIONS ABOUT PROPOLIS

How much should I take?

Authorities differ on this issue. Dr McEwan,[1] the allergy specialist referred to earlier, recommends a minimum dose of 1.5g, i.e. 1500 milligrams, of refined propolis per day, and other authorities confirm this. One of the reasons he claims propolis sometimes has a poor reputation is because not enough is taken. Dr Murat[2] suggested between 25–30g should be taken over a single treatment period lasting around ten days. This roughly equates to 3g per day twice, the dosage suggested by Dr. McEwan's. However, Russian doctors with many years' experience in using propolis, are known to prescribe up to 9g of propolis a day for some serious conditions, without any particular side effects. As we saw earlier, in the section on ME, those with seriously compromised immune systems were taking up to 12g per day.[3] These amounts would seem excessive unless they are being prescribed for a serious condition. Faced with the onset of a particular problem—flu, cough, cold, respiratory problems—it may be appropriate to take a larger quantity initially and then reduce the regular dose over the following period.

How should I take it?

I have already described the variety of ways in which you can take propolis, the most common being as capsules, tablets or liquid. Probably the best way to take propolis, however, is raw, straight from the hive. In chewing propolis your salivary juices slowly extract the active elements from the raw material. Dr Felix Murat[4] recommends: 'Chewing it in its pure form for mouth, nose and throat ailments or for broncho-pulmonary infections, the recommended dosage is three grams daily.' He recommends that raw propolis should be chewed for about half an hour, until it becomes soft, at which point it can be swallowed. Unfortunately you have to be sure that the source is pure and free from contamination and this is not always easy.

By far the vast majority of people who take propolis regularly use capsules or tablets. However, consumers are increasingly choosing propolis liquid because they believe it acts more quickly. Propolis in liquid is more instantly bio-available. Asthma sufferers in particular have noted that if propolis liquid is taken as soon as symptoms appear it can ward off an attack.

If you are using propolis externally, again you have a variety of forms you can choose from. Generally, propolis creams contain only a small amount of propolis, usually between one–two per cent. Ointments can contain more, while propolis liquids can contain up to 25 per cent refined propolis.

When should I take it?

This partly depends on what you are using propolis for. It is probably best to spread your dose over the day. Propolis is best taken on an empty stomach,[5] particularly if you are looking to address a problem connected with the gut or stomach, such as *Candida* or an inflammatory condition.

It is probably best not to take propolis last thing at night. Some people report difficulties with sleeping if propolis is taken too late at night although it can depend on your overall temperament whether propolis keeps you awake or sends you to sleep.[6]

How long should I take it for?

Many people take 500mg of propolis per day simply to stay well and to keep their immune system in trim. As with any natural medicines, however, it is recommended that you rest your body from it every six to eight weeks for perhaps a week at a time.

When fighting a particular problem Dr Murat and others recommend a course of treatment of up to ten days followed by a break for up to a week unless the problem reoccurs.[7] Clearly, the dose and treatment period is going to vary according to the nature of the problem and its seriousness.

Can I take it with orthodox medicines?

We have seen earlier research that illustrates how propolis can improve the effectiveness of antibiotics.[8] Dr Murat suggests that propolis may be taken with antibiotics and other medicines but only on the advice of your physician or medical herbalist. There do not appear to be any problems relating to the interaction of propolis and orthodox medicines. The evidence does suggest that propolis improves your body's metabolism and boosts its immune system. Some patients undergoing chemotherapy for cancer, for instance, report that taking propolis before and during the treatment radically reduces some unpleasant side effects of chemical therapy—ulcerated mouth, for example. However, more research is required before this area can be properly understood.

Are there any side effects?

People have been taking propolis, as a medicine for around 3,000 years and nowhere in the literature is there mention of any serious or toxic side effects. However, environmental pollution has introduced some new concerns to our understanding of natural products over the last few years. Lead, pesticide and radioactivity pollution, have all been recognised as potential problems over the last few years. However, reputable manufacturers either remove these elements or routinely test for them.

One problem has traditionally been associated with propolis and is referred to frequently in scientific literature. Roughly one in every thousand people is allergic to propolis. The cause of the allergy is still unknown. Many people associate all bee products with allergies, principally because of the reputation of pollen and honey, but as propolis, especially when it is refined, is composed of almost pure resin collected from trees, it should contain neither pollen nor honey. Some manufacturers do include pollen in their propolis capsules but this should be noted on the label.

Allergic responses occur far less often when propolis is taken internally than when it is applied externally. This is ironic as propolis, as we have seen, has been used successfully to treat asthma, hay fever and skin problems.

Again, caution should be exercised when you first take propolis. An allergic response can show itself as a reddening of the skin and itchiness. If you are using propolis to treat skin problems like psoriasis or eczema then a patch test is advisable first.

Excessive use of propolis can sometimes cause diarrhoea.

Can children take it?

According to Dr Murat[9] a child's dose should be half that of an adult and the treatment, however it is taken, should begin with smaller doses and gradually built up.

How do I know which product to buy?

Make sure when buying propolis that the amount of propolis contained in each capsule, tablet or liquid dose, etc. is clearly stated. Virtually all manufacturers now sell refined and not raw propolis. Five hundred milligrams of refined propolis is very roughly equal to 1 gram of raw. So if on the label it says: *These capsules contain the equivalent of 1000 milligrams of raw propolis*, it probably means it actually contains between 350–500g of refined propolis. Most reputable manufacturers will now refer to the content of refined propolis.

In the UK you can look out for the HFMA (Health Food Manufacturers Association) propolis specification mark. (See Appendix 1—HFMA Propolis Specification). This should mean that you can rely on the fact that this product has been tested and meets the minimum specification laid down for propolis including a minimum level of bioflavonoids. (See Setting Standards.)

Can I buy organic propolis?

Organic propolis is available but as yet the quantities are very small. The problem is that bees can forage for over three miles in any direction from the hive, which means that all land must be free from pesticides, herbicides, etc. within a three-mile radius of the hives. Unless a manufacturer can show that propolis was produced from bees in the middle of such an extremely large certified organic farm, the propolis is not organic. The majority of propolis used by commercial manufacturers comes from China where few environmental regulations apply.

NON-MEDICINAL USES OF PROPOLIS

Whilst propolis is associated most commonly with the treatment of illness, it has been used for a wide variety of purposes including varnishes, cosmetics, wine and in food.

Varnishes—from sledges to Stradivarius

The preservative properties of propolis have been recognised for centuries and propolis has been used as a component of a variety of products designed to prevent rusting or decay or to maintain the brilliance and colour of pieces treated. For example, older beekeepers would dip their metal tools in a propolis liquid to prevent rusting, while Siberians and Mongolians were known to soak their sledges in a propolis-and-turpentine mixture in order to protect them against the intense cold.[10]

Russians still use a propolis varnish to treat and preserve furniture. The varnish is composed of two parts propolis mixed with five parts linseed oil and one part wax. The mixture is gently heated to melt the wax and blend the constituents after which it must be left to settle and mature. Items of furniture are dipped in the varnish and left to dry before being polished.

Perhaps the most famous use of propolis varnish was its use during the seventeenth and eighteenth centuries by master violin-makers including Stradivarius and Guarneri.[11] It is thought that the propolis-and-wax mix provided just the right blend of soft and hard qualities able to preserve the violin yet keep it supple. Some have suggested that the varnish may also have been responsible for the beautiful colour and tone of some of these instruments. Manufacturers of stringed instruments still use propolis varnish today.

An alcohol extract of propolis was also used traditionally to maintain and enhance the lustre of gold and silver as well as in treating leather goods.

Felix Murat[12] reports on its use as an additive to make paint glossy. Propolis is again dissolved in linseed oil and then mixed with any oil-based paint in a ratio of one to five. As well as giving the paint a glossy texture the paint apparently also lasts longer.

Propolis and tobacco—breath freshener to mind-expander

In 1989 a patent was taken out in the USA for a 'propolis-containing, resin-based chewing tobacco'![13] Chewing tobacco is still popular in the US and propolis was added to the tobacco, as a breath freshener and to reduce the throat and stomach irritation that often accompanies tobacco chewing.

Again, Felix Murat[14] explores at some length the effect of smoking tobacco which has been soaked in propolis—reporting that it acts both as a stimulant and as a tranquilliser. Of the 17 participants in his experimental group who tried smoking it, six said it had 'an exhilarating effect.' In a further four subjects it induced sleep, in two psychic experiences, and five said it had no effect at all. However, when stronger solutions of propolis were used, it apparently induced altered states of awareness similar to those of marijuana, another resin.

According to Murat, propolis has a tranquillising or stimulating effect depending on the current state of mind of the user. If the user is stressed, then the propolis can exacerbate that condition and similarly, if the user is relaxed he will further relax. Bearing in mind the current interest in the medicinal use of marijuana to treat multiple sclerosis, it may be that Murat's experiments warrant further attention. Propolis, like marijuana, has strong anaesthetic properties and may therefore have a role to play in the pain control of some conditions following appropriate research.

Propolis in wine, brandy and fortified spirits

Propolis has been used to fortify both wine and spirits. In some Eastern European countries propolis wine is commercially available and in Russia you can purchase vodka and brandy containing small quantities of propolis. We have seen how another resin, from the poplar tree, is added to retsina wine in Greece.

Mead, a honey liqueur no doubt containing elements of propolis, has of course been made in Europe since medieval times. If you want to try this yourself, you can add a small quantity (about a quarter of an ounce) of finely ground propolis to a bottle of wine (preferably organic), leaving it to dissolve in the wine over a week to ten days, gently shaking the bottle periodically. Home wine makers can add the propolis prior to the bottling stage. You can do the same of course with bottles of spirits—vodka, whisky or brandy. For many, propolis has a notoriously unpleasant taste—clearly our ancestors found a way round this problem.

Propolis drinks

The market for energy drinks in the West and particularly in Japan is vast and a number of manufacturers have taken the opportunity of creating specialist propolis drinks.

Propolis in food

Propolis can be added to other foods in a variety of ways. If you make your own bread then instead of adding sugar you can blend a little finely ground propolis with honey. You will need to add extra yeast to the mixture as the propolis slows down the activity of yeast.

Propolis vinegar can be used to make a dressing for salad. The vinegar effectively masks the strong taste of propolis. Again, you will need a fine powder which is added to the vinegar each time you use it, in the same proportions as you might add salt or pepper.

CHAPTER 8

Propolis and Animals

Not surprisingly, given its success in treating human disease, propolis has also been used to treat both farm and domestic animals. Once again, much of the research has been conducted in Eastern Europe, particularly in Russia, although increasing interest is now been shown in the West.

The importance of propolis in the USSR for treating animals was emphasised in a 1978 report from its Ministry of Agriculture[1] on the use of propolis in veterinary science. In that report propolis was recommended in various forms—liquid extracts, emulsions and ointments—for the treatment of burns, superficial wounds, abscesses, skin diseases and mastitis. It was recommended particularly for young animals with, for example, digestive disturbances or bronchopneumonia. The suggested dose was 3ml per kilo live weight.

In 1989 a Chinese delegation[2] to the XXXIInd International Congress of Apiculture reported on work it had done in the veterinary field since they had first been alerted to the use of propolis at an earlier congress in 1975. They told the Congress that they had conducted many experiments exploring the bacteriostatic potential of propolis in treating animals. Propolis had been found to be useful in treating domestic animals affected by seventeen different pathogenic species. These included *Staphylococcus aureus, Streptococcus equi, Erysipelotbrix busiopathia, Pasteurelia suispeptica, Pasteurella bovisseptica, Salmonella abortus-equi, Salmonella cholerae Suis, Salmonella pullorum, Salmonella gallinarum, Bacillus coli, Listerella monocytogenies, Salmonella paratyphi A, Salmonell typhi, Pseudomonas aeruginosa, Streptococcus B.* and *Shigella flexner*.

Commercial animal husbandry faces a crisis, of which BSE is

only the tip of the iceberg. The gross overuse of antibiotics, as growth promoters and to treat disease, has left veterinary science, as with human medical science, nowhere to go. Slowly but surely, interest is turning to natural and herbal medicine and propolis undoubtedly has a big part to play as the review of the animal research below shows.

TREATMENT OF CATTLE

Researchers in Moscow[3] treated 28 cows with mastitis (an acute inflammation of the udder normally treated with antibiotics). The cows were put on a diet and the infected teats treated with a propolis emulsion. Seven ml of the propolis emulsion was introduced directly into the teat three times every 24 hours for eight days. Apart from one case of purulent mastitis the bacterial count in all the cows fell sharply after one or two treatments. On average the mastitis was cured in between five–seven days depending on its type and severity. What is interesting about this research is not only the effectiveness of the propolis treatment but that milking did not stop, as it must when antibiotics are used, and that virtually full milk production was restored in all but two of the cows.

In 1985[4] and 1989[5] Polish researchers successfully used propolis to treat mastitis in 146 cows. The treatment was completely successful in 125 cases, including all cases caused by *Candida albicans* and the vast majority of the cases caused by *E.coli, Staphylococci* and *Streptococci*. The researchers also noted that propolis was effective against micro-organisms that had become resistant to the antibiotics then currently in use.

Experiments were conducted at the Moscow Veterinary Institute,[6] both on uterine sections taken from cows and on live cows, to explore the effect of propolis in stimulating uterine contractions. Propolis was found to increase the number and intensity of the contractions—a piece of research of obvious importance in ensuring live healthy birth of calves.

Research at the Kazan Veterinary Institute[7] in 1971 illustrated how propolis when used with copper cobalt TKP on animals carrying paratyphoid antigens, significantly increased the animal's immunogenesis and activated the production of anti-bodies and phagocytosis. Similar research was undertaken in 1972 at the Kirov Institute, USSR,[8] when propolis was used in conjunction with a vaccine to immunise calves against paratyphoid. The propolis, it was found, stimulated the creation of agglutinins, which the body needs to fight the virus.

In 1988 investigators at Brno University, Czechoslovakia,[9] used an extract of propolis to treat injured teeth in calves and claimed that it accelerated the healing process.

In 1990 Italian researchers[10] treated fungal infections in cattle with a 10 per cent propolis in petroleum jelly solution. Again, they claimed the treatment accelerated the healing process.

One of the most interesting and potentially important uses of propolis in animal husbandry came out of a 1987 project in Hungary.[11] A 20 per cent extract of propolis in between 2–5ml doses was added to the morning and evening milk feed of young calves. The calves fed on the propolis supplement not only had less incidences of diarrhoea or scouring than the control group but also gained weight faster than the controls. At a time where so-called growth promoters, often containing antibiotics, are facing closer scrutiny by the regulators, it may be that propolis can provide an effective natural alternative with considerable added benefit in terms of overall health for the animal.

Aujeszky's disease is a virus, which can cause forms of paralysis in cattle and horses. In 1979 research at the Kazan Veterinary Institute, USSR,[12] tested a propolis treatment on chicks infected with the virus. Apart from those with the heaviest infections all treated simultaneously with an aqueous emulsion of propolis survived.

In 1999 Korean researchers[13] reported on the use of propolis as a feed additive on the treatment and prevention of neonatal diarrhoea in calves. Twenty calves were artificially infected with *E.coli*, a major cause of neonatal diarrhoea. Propolis was shown to be equally as effective as enrofloxacin. The researchers felt that propolis could provide an environmentally sound alternative to antibiotics in treating this problem.

TREATMENT OF PIGS

Aujeszky's disease also affects pigs and was once endemic in the UK. Russian researchers[14] found in 1976 that pigs vaccinated against Aujeszky's disease typically developed the necessary antibodies seven days after injection. However, if the suckling pigs were injected simultaneously with the equivalent of 5–10mgs of propolis as an emulsion, then this increased the number of antibodies produced by between three–four times.

Similar research at the famous Kazan Veterinary Institute, USSR, in 1977[15] repeated the experiment with older pigs. When the animals were slaughtered two–three weeks after vaccination it was observed that those pigs which had been injected solely with the vaccine showed significant damage to a number of their internal organs, whereas those treated simultaneously with propolis did not. Furthermore, the pigs given the additional propolis treatment were found to have increased their formation of antibodies by two–three times more than the controls as well as having an enhanced production of plasmacytes in the lymphoidal tissue of the spleen.

One of the most remarkable studies relates to the use of propolis as a feed supplement for small pigs. A Romanian study in 1983[16] showed that when small amounts of propolis were included in the diet of piglets, those piglets both gained more weight and ate less food than the control group. Food consumption was down by a huge 29 per cent compared with the control group. The researchers believed the reason for this lay in the ability of propolis to prevent digestive disorders, so increasing the effective digestion of available food.

The use of antibiotics and other growth promoters are increasingly restricted in the pig industry in the UK and elsewhere. Two research projects have recently begun in North Yorkshire, England. Pig breeders and vets committed to a more natural and, in one case organic, regime are beginning to explore the potential of propolis. They are looking at its use as a general health promoter, as a growth promoter and as a specific treatment for problems which affect young pigs, in particular scouring and pneumonia.

TREATMENT OF POULTRY

The Romanian researchers referred to above also showed that propolis as a feed supplement was of marked benefit to poultry. The results were equally dramatic, with pullets putting on more weight than the controls despite eating 14 per cent less food.

Earlier research at the University of Palma, Italy,[17] had come to much the same conclusion. By putting propolis in the food of battery hens, at a ratio of around 30 parts per million, they achieved an increase in egg laying of 6.07 per cent, egg weight of 1.27 per cent, food utilization of 5.46 per cent and an overall weight increase in the pullets of 6.40 per cent. The researchers also noted that there were no adverse effects on the colour of the yoke or on the death rate of the hens.

TREATMENT OF SHEEP

Romanian research[18] in 1974 described the treatment of 12 sheep with serious purulent wounds. Apparently, initially, neither of two commercially available antibiotic powders nor propolis had any bactericidal effects on these wounds. However, after 12–14 days the propolis treatment showed a strong healing effect.

During 1985 and 1986 Uruguayan agricultural researchers[19] used propolis to treat sheep which, in previous years, had shown a very high incidence of foot rot. They applied propolis to the feet of 80 adult rams. During the two years when the animals were treated around 20 per cent of the animals showed signs of infection but none of the sheep became clinical cases.

We have already referred to a series of remarkable experiments carried out on sheep and dogs in Bulgaria in 1973, testing the natural anaesthetic effects of propolis.[20] Propolis extract was used in the same way, as an anaesthetic prior to surgical operations. The anaesthetic effect of propolis was observed after two–five minutes of local application and lasted for about 45 minutes. The researcher claims he saw no difference between the anaesthetic effect of propolis and that of novocaine. However, the effect of propolis was slower than that of novocaine. As far as I am aware these experiments have never been repeated.

TREATMENT OF RABBITS AND RATS

Two research projects carried out in the mid 1980s at the University of Havana, in Cuba,[21] illustrated the anti-parasitic properties of propolis. In these experiments rabbits were artificially infected with a number of parasites, including the protozoan parasite *Eimeria*. In one experiment the rabbits were then treated with a two–three per cent solution of propolis administered in their drinking water. Over a period of four weeks the rabbits showed an average of 80 per cent reduction in the number of *Eimeria* occysts excreted. A later experiment compared propolis with some conventional sulphur-based products. The coccidiostatic effect of the propolis was found to be superior to that of the sulphonamides.[22]

Rats and other small animals have, as we have seen earlier been used extensively to test a range of the pharmacological activities of propolis. In a Japanese study[23] in 1990 propolis was tested on rats artificially infected with the bacteria which cause dental caries. The propolis was found to have both anti-microbial effects and to inhibit the synthesis and destructive activity of sugars involved in dental caries. No toxic effects were observed on the growth of the rats.

Much of the research quoted here is now some years old but it is none the less indicative of the wide range of benefits that can be achieved using propolis. In many cases propolis is shown to be more effective than synthetic alternatives. Obviously more work needs to be done but the time is right. Farmers concerned about spiralling costs and decreasing effectiveness of synthetic drugs as well as the mounting restrictions on their use are ready to give nature a chance again. One imagines, however, that the research that will excite farmers most will be in the use of propolis as a 'growth promoter'. More weight gain with less food could be a salvation for many food producers in the UK who currently face extremely difficult times. These aspects of animal research, more than any other, illustrate the powerful holistic effect of propolis. Put simply, the animals put on more weight with less food because their whole system is functioning in a more effective and healthy way. Whether or not the commercial use of propolis in this area adds up remains to be seen. However, what farmers will need to bear in mind is not just the simple weight gained by animals but the overall improvement in health and consequent saving in routine treatment costs for a variety of separate health problems.

PETS AND PERFORMANCE ANIMALS

The last few years have seen a huge increase in the use of natural products to treat domestic animals. When propolis became popular in the UK in the mid-nineties, reports began to trickle through that users were treating their pets with it too, and for many of the same reasons they themselves were taking it: eczema, joint problems, respiratory problems, wounds and infections. One dog breeder in North Yorkshire, England, reported that persistent ear infections common to his particular breed had begun to clear up when treated with propolis tincture, while eczema, again common in his highly-bred animals, responded quickly to treatment with propolis cream. Overall fitness of the animals improved and in particular their coats became glossier.

The best way to administer propolis to pet animals is to mix the tincture, or powder from emptied capsules or crushed tablets with its food. Where treatment is required externally, simply apply in the same way as for human use.

Using propolis to treat hedgehogs made national news in the UK in 1996. A hedgehog sanctuary in Lincolnshire, UK, had been asked to treat a hedgehog which had been brutally burnt and sprayed with paint. The spineless and scarred hedgehog, Kevin, was treated solely with propolis liquid and cream, made a full recovery and was eventually released back into the wild. The sanctuary is often asked to treat hedgehogs which are accidentally burnt or injured by unsuspecting gardeners. In each case they now use propolis to treat the burns and wounds.

One bee product company in America has developed a product containing propolis, along with pollen and royal jelly, especially for pet birds. The product can be introduced into the bird's food. Up to a teaspoonful per day is recommended for large birds. Again, these highly-bred birds benefit from propolis, being less susceptible to avian viruses and generally fitter and with shinier coats, an important factor for show birds.

Owners of performance animals too are turning to propolis as a way of improving their fitness and performance. One racehorse trainer in the North of England found that adding a mix of propolis and pollen to his horses feed meant these sometimes delicate animals were less susceptible to the viruses which are common in racing stables. Animals fed this supplement were less likely to go down with the equine equivalent of our coughs, colds and flu viruses.

In the US propolis and other bee products have been in regular use on the racetrack for many years. One manufacturer claims it can 'aid your horse's recovery from nagging conditions and help keep him healthy for that upcoming competition.'

CHAPTER 9

Propolis—The Impact of Commercial Exploitation

With the blossoming of interest in natural medicine in the 1980s and 1990s one can see that propolis was a success story waiting to happen. However, despite a short-lived renaissance in UK health stores in the 1970s, by the early 1990s all that remained of it was a few bottles of propolis tincture tucked away in the back of health food shops. But in 1994 the position of propolis in the UK was to change dramatically, following publication of a piece about it in a national newspaper.

PROPOLIS HITS THE HEADLINES

In 1993, a national UK health magazine[1] published a piece about propolis and its properties alongside details of a new company formed by two propolis enthusiasts in the North of England. In the article they reviewed the price of propolis per gram available to consumers from a variety of manufacturers. The propolis in the products produced by the new company was costing consumers around £1 per gram, whereas most companies were charging significantly more, with one company effectively charging £75 per gram. Propolis slowly began to get a reputation amongst the health conscious as a useful product.

In early 1994 a journalist who had found propolis useful in treating his own chronic asthma decided to write about it in his newspaper, a paper with a readership of over four million people.[2] In the piece he referred to its use in treating asthma, arthritis and eczema. Within a couple of months of publication, virtually every health food store in the country was selling propolis products. The natural health press, always on the look out for a new product story, took to propolis with a vengeance and countless articles appeared over the next 18 months. The headline writers had a field day. Propolis was labelled as 'The Bees Knees', as a 'Bee line to health', 'Bee Positive', 'Praise Bee' and manufacturers were 'buzzing with success'. But this high-profile exposure and commercial success for propolis brought in its wake a number of problems.

LEAD CONTAMINATION

Late in 1994, at the height of the media interest in propolis, one brand on sale in London was found by local Trading Standards Officers (the UK consumer protection body) to contain higher than permitted levels of lead.

Propolis, like most natural health products, is sold as a food, and not as a medicine, and as such, is governed by the UK food regulations. Under these regulations, no food may be sold for human consumption if it contains more than one part per million lead. (1 ppm). The product analysed contained 1500 ppm, still a relatively small amount bearing in mind the very small quantities consumers were ingesting, but hugely over the permitted levels for foods. Other propolis products on the market were also tested and all of them were found to contain lead above the permitted levels.

At one point the UK Ministry of Agriculture considered banning the sale of propolis altogether. Instead, it and the Department of Health instructed all the companies then selling propolis in the UK to withdraw all products from the market containing more than 1 ppm.

Many felt that this was unfair treatment. The food regulations, it was argued, were designed to regulate the levels of lead in food products consumed in quantity. Propolis, it was argued, was consumed in very small quantities, each capsule containing a maximum of 500mgs of propolis in total. Indeed, some food products—some fish products and for some reason tomato paste—were specifically allowed by the food laws to contain up to 15 ppm lead and licensed medicines were allowed to contain up to 40 ppm.

The problem for European and American propolis manufacturers

TRANSACTION RECORD

THE ORIGINAL
POQUITO MÁS
BAJA TACO STAND®

CARD TYPE:Visa
No.:************0038
ENTRY:SWIPED
AUTHORIZATION:016175
STORE #:1
TERMINAL:2
REFERENCE:735655

PURCHASE $18.59

THANK YOU
MAY 18,2010 16:17:11
Server's name : yesica

CUSTOMER COPY

was that very few sources of raw propolis could be found that did not contain more than the permitted levels of lead. Most Chinese propolis at the time contained around 2– 300 ppm; Russian propolis had lower levels of between 10–50 ppm and European propolis, depending on the source, between 10–30 ppm.

Manufacturers soon realised that if propolis was to remain on the market they would have to find novel ways of refining it which removed lead to the permitted levels whilst retaining the wholeness and integrity of the product. A number of companies took up this challenge and some of the methods developed are discussed below.

COLLECTING PROPOLIS

According to Ochi in 1981[3] and Andrich in 1987[4] a single colony of bees produces between ten and 300 grams (between ⅓ ounce to ten ounces) of propolis per year. The exact quantity varies according to the type of bee, the tree and plant resources available, the climate and the method of collection. Many beekeepers report much higher quantities than this.

Only a small proportion of the propolis bees produce is commercially harvested. Many beekeepers still see propolis as a nuisance rather than as a powerful medicine and therefore a commercial product. These beekeepers are more likely to choose bees which produce less rather than more propolis, if it means their principal tasks of collecting honey or breeding queens is made easier.

Nevertheless the annual amount of raw propolis harvested worldwide is thought to be around 300–400 tonnes. Assuming each hive produces an average of 300g per colony, per year, this equates to an astonishing 1.3 million hives from which propolis is harvested in any one year.

By far the largest commercial producer of propolis is China but other significant producers include the old Soviet Union, Europe, South America, Australia New Zealand and the USA. As the commercial profile of propolis has increased so other countries have begun to explore cost-effective ways of harvesting propolis, often as a way of adding value to subsistence agriculture systems. In Africa, where propolis has traditionally been used medicinally and for other purposes, collection systems are now being developed, as they are India and the Far East.

The world price for raw untreated propolis, depending on quality, is currently around $15–$20 per kilo if purchased in tonne quantities. In the 1970s, when propolis made its first commercial appearance in the West, Dr Aagard Lund, in Denmark, was paying American beekeepers $200 per kilo.

At current prices $20 buys the annual production of around four hives. At this price, the propolis has to be collected, sorted, cleaned, brought, often long distances, to regional collection points, weighed, packed and transported, sometimes halfway around the world, to major refiners in the West or Japan. Clearly, propolis is only worth collecting if you have access to low-cost labour.

Traditionally, propolis has been collected by scraping it from the entrance, walls, frames and covers of the hive. This method—still practised widely—can result in considerable contamination from wood particles, paint, wax and other debris. Marletto[5] noted that propolis collected from the cover or top of frames was cleaner than that collected near the entrance.

Beekeepers committed to collecting propolis commercially are increasingly turning to specialised propolis traps. These traps are essentially screens containing a series of small holes placed on the top of the hive. The bees identify these holes and cracks as a threat to the integrity of the hive and are compelled to fill them with propolis.

The simplest propolis trap is made up of a wooden frame the size of a horizontal cross-section of the hive, with a nylon fly screen drawn across it. This screen is inserted at the top of the hive underneath the top board, which is propped open slightly. Other purpose-built traps involve semi-rigid plastic sheets with rows of slots in them, which the bees fill in order to seal up the hive. (See illustrations 1, 2 and 3). When the traps are full, they are removed and placed in a freezer. When chilled the propolis becomes brittle and can easily be removed by flexing the plastic sheets or bending the fly screen material. Collecting propolis this way produces both the best quality and cleanest propolis.

Not all propolis, particularly that which is used to cap the cells or is built into the comb itself, is accessible by either of the above methods. The Chinese, noted for their ingenuity and thriftiness,

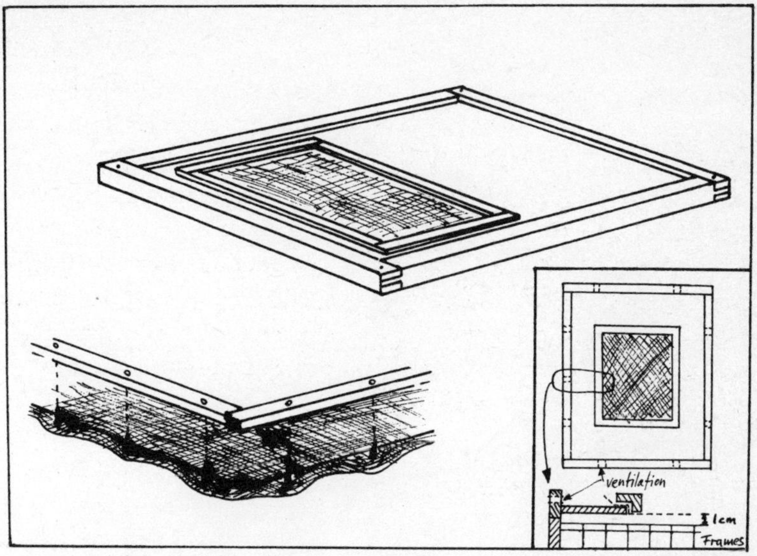

A simple to make propolis trap made from nylon fly or mosquito screen. The screen can be easily removed and replaced with a new one during the harvest. Taken from Krell, R. Value added products from beekeeping, FAO, Bulletin 124, 1996.

use a simple method for extracting this. Following honey extraction, the empty comb and cappings are left to melt in the sun on a sloping surface. The wax runs off first leaving behind the propolis and any other debris.

None of these methods lend themselves to industrial-style production and the propolis harvested in this way is hard won. However, as the commercial demand for high quality, clean propolis grows, we may expect more effective, but hopefully not more exploitative, methods to be developed.

EXTRACTING AND REFINING PROPOLIS

Probably one of the most effective ways of extracting the active components of propolis is to chew it! Your salivary juices slowly release the bittersweet anaesthetic quality of the propolis which, after a few minutes chewing, turns into the consistency of a waxy chewing gum. Providing the propolis is clean and from an environmentally safe area this is an ideal way of taking propolis

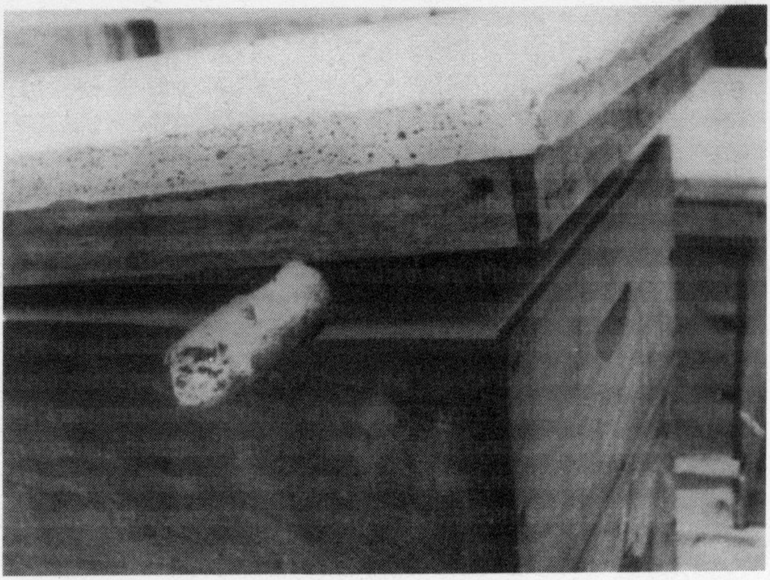

Four sheets are placed on the top super with wider sides of the hole facing down with bee space (1 cm) bet sheets and frame tops. The cover of the hive is then left open to increase ventilation and let light in. This stimulates the bees to seal the slots with propolis. Taken from Krell, R. Value added products of beekeeping, FAO, Bulletin 124. 1996.

and in particular of treating mouth ulcers and dental problems.

Traditionally, the most popular way of extracting and preserving propolis is to soak a few ounces of raw propolis in alcohol—vodka in Russia—and then sieve out any physical debris. In many Eastern European markets small balls of propolis are still commonly offered for sale with other bee products for just this purpose. (See chapter 10: Making Your Own Medicines.)

Inevitably, commercial demands for large-scale quantities of propolis and the increasing demands of safety and regulatory bodies have led to increasing sophistication of the extraction process, and to the development of novel extraction techniques. In particular, the problem with lead has sharply focussed the attention of all manufacturers on ways of overcoming the impact of environmental pollution in general—heavy metals, pesticides and radioactivity. This has meant that over the last few years refining technology has improved radically. Unfortunately, in some

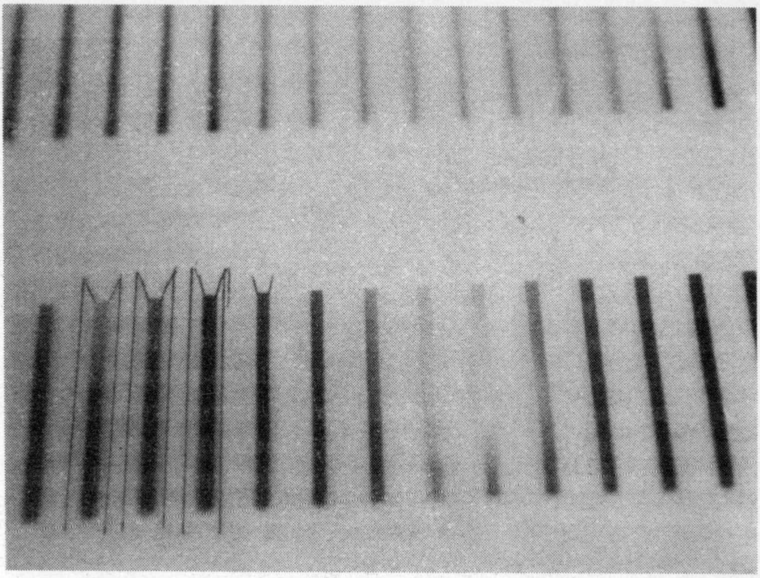

3 mm plastic sheets with rows of slots, 2 mm on one side and 4 mm on the other side which the bees are compelled to close. Taken from Krell, R. Value added products of beekeeping, FAO, Bulletin 124, 1996.

cases this has also resulted in propolis being over-refined, which can undermine or even destroy the integrity of the product and impair its holistic and synergistic function.

The choice of extraction solvents is affected both by cost—alcohol in most places attracts duty whereas propylene glycol and water do not—as well as the intended end use for the product. For example, cosmetic manufacturers may prefer a propylene glycol extract because it mixes more easily when preparing creams or lotions. Propylene glycol is also preferred for oral and nasal sprays because it stays in place longer—it does not evaporate as quickly as alcohol. However, propylene glycol is not particularly recommended for internal use and research has shown that too much propylene glycol can cause fits and heart problems.

Using alcohol to extract propolis

Most commercial refining processes still use alcohol, usually ethanol, as the preferred solvent to extract and refine propolis. We have seen from the research data that EEP (Ethanol Extracted Propolis) appears more than any other preparation in pharmacological and clinical tests.

If the propolis is for internal human consumption then it is important that the purest alcohol is used. Denatured alcohol, that is alcohol which has had chemicals added to prevent it being drunk, should not normally be used as the chemicals added to denature the product can have toxic effects which can sometimes be fatal when taken internally.

In general, the higher the concentration of alcohol used, the more effective and complete the extraction will be. Non-commercial users recommend that the propolis be soaked in the alcohol for two or three weeks before filtration to maximise the extraction of the key 'active' elements. Soaking the propolis for longer than this apparently does not increase the amount extracted. Large-scale manufacturers working with batches of up to one ton or more often use heat to help 'dissolve' the propolis and speed the process of extraction. This initial heat also acts to separate the wax from the resin, which can be taken off prior to any filtration process. However, as little heat as possible should be used as this can change, even destroy, the synergistic effect of the propolis. Continued high temperatures are most damaging, changing or destroying the biochemical structure of the bioflavonoids.

Heat also aids the filtration process. The propolis liquid is pumped through a very fine filter, with holes as little as 4 microns across. This removes not only particles of debris in the propolis but non-dissolved particles of lead. This process, is however, not able to remove volatile leads, i.e. organic lead compounds, which dissolve in alcohol, and neither can it remove pesticides and other chemical contaminants.

New technology has been developed by a number of companies to deal with both these problems using CO_2 (carbon dioxide) extraction and ion exchange technology.

Depending on what finished products are required, it may be necessary to remove the solvent from the propolis. In the laboratory or in small-scale manufacturing this can be done by leaving the alcohol to evaporate or by applying heat. However, this is a laborious and potentially dangerous operation. In commercial processes alcohol is removed using vacuum drying, freeze-drying or spray drying. Vacuum drying speeds up the process because lower temperatures are necessary under vacuum for the alcohol to evaporate. The process is also safer as the evaporation takes place in a sealed vessel. It is possible with vacuum drying to remove the alcohol entirely leaving a solid dry, dark resin, which can be milled and powdered, and which is used principally for producing tablets and capsules.

Using propylene glycol to extract propolis

The extraction process using propylene glycol is similar to that of alcohol. However, propylene glycol is more viscous than alcohol and will not dissolve the same concentrations of propolis. Propylene glycol will dissolve 10 per cent propolis by weight, whereas alcohol will dissolve 50 per cent propolis.

It is also more difficult to remove the solvent if this is required. High temperatures are required to evaporate propylene glycol, which runs the risk of damaging the product.

Using water to extract propolis

Water-extracted propolis is produced by either soaking propolis in water or immersing it in boiling water. Obviously this process extracts only those elements which are water-soluble. Whilst these extracts have been shown to have some of the same anti-bacterial and anti-fungal properties as EEP it is generally recognised that their biological effect is not as potent as the ethanol-extracted material.

Using oils to extract propolis

Finally, oils—peach oil, almond oil, olive oil, etc.—can be used to extract propolis. This is a very slow process and does not lend itself to commercial production. It is suited to small-scale manufacturing of creams. (See Chapter 9 Making Your Own Medicines.)

Water-soluble and water-dispersible propolis

Increasingly, consumers are demanding both alcohol and propylene glycol-free products. In Muslim countries in particular, alcohol is specifically prohibited and in Japan, for example, propylene glycol is banned in all but extremely low concentrations. Alcohol-based products are not recommended for pregnant women, children and for the treatment of some conditions, i.e. stomach ulcers and eye and skin problems.

The market for a water-soluble extract of propolis has been recognised by a number of researchers and manufacturers.

A Bulgarian patent[9] describes a process in which an alcohol-extracted propolis is dried and mixed with L-lysine solution at 50–60°C (122–140°F). The solution is then freeze-dried, producing a yellow-brown propolis powder. So far, no published research has been carried out on the impact of the L-lysine solution on the active elements of propolis.

An Italian company has patented a micro-encapsulating process, which they claim produces a 'water-dispersible' rather than water-soluble product, which they say improves the bioavailability of the propolis.[10] Research carried out by the company into the microbiological activity of a mouthwash using this preparation showed positive results but this work has not so far been published.

An UK patent takes a different approach, using a colloidal mill to reduce the particulate size of propolis to one where when dry, it can be suspended in a variety of non-alcoholic liquids. Propolis products in maple syrup have been developed using this technique, which the company claims improves bioavailability as well as making propolis liquid more palatable, particularly for children. One disadvantage of this non-alcoholic process is that preservatives may be required if the carrier solution is not naturally preserving.

POPULARITY EQUALS POOR QUALITY

In the six months following the 1994 media exposure of propolis, sales boomed. For several months, propolis was the fastest selling natural health supplement in the UK, outstripping many of the usual best sellers.

In 1994 the value of the market for propolis products in the UK went from around £100,000 per year to between £2–3 million per year. The market was flooded with propolis products, not just from the UK but from Europe and America. Where there had been three or four brands available to consumers, soon there were 20 or more. All of them, of course, claimed to be the purest, the highest concentration and the best value for money. The problem was that, far from being the best, some products on the market were in fact of very poor quality and in some cases were not even propolis at all.

For example, a number of products imported from the US claimed to be 5:1 extracts of propolis produced by 'state of the art technology'. This means that 5 grams of raw propolis were refined to produce 1 gram of pure finished product. These products were presented to consumers at very low prices, so low in fact that they could not possibly have been produced for the price charged. At the time, one of these 5:1 products was tested in a leading German laboratory with many years of experience and understanding of propolis. It came back from the laboratory with the comment 'no known properties of propolis.'

The problem for consumers was that they had no effective way of discriminating between good quality products and fake ones. No simple test then existed that would enable Trading Standards officers to determine whether a particular propolis product was good, bad or even authentic, let alone effective.

The consumer protection authorities, as we have seen, are primarily concerned with the enforcement of food regulations, for example, whether the product contains over the permitted levels of lead. In fact, many of the 5:1 products did very well on the lead test but only because, in some cases, they were not propolis at all. Some products tested turned out to be pure cocoa powder!

This problem is not peculiar to propolis. The same thing has happened to other natural products which have become suddenly and dramatically popular. Poor quality or even counterfeit products at very competitive prices flood the market before either consumers or regulatory bodies can get a true understanding of how to evaluate and judge them. When this happens it tarnishes the image of the products themselves and the natural health movement in general. Consumers find that the products do not work as they had expected and are then perhaps less inclined to believe in a natural approach in the future.

Addressing this problem for propolis has been long and tortuous. It has required the co-operation of all the major UK manufacturers, research to identify and quantify some of the key biochemicals in propolis, the development of simple cost-effective testing procedures and the establishment and supervision of a quality mark which consumers can understand and recognise.

SETTING STANDARDS FOR PROPOLIS

Inevitably, it is difficult to set a fixed standard for a natural product which varies so much according to climate, flora, season, etc. The earliest standards were developed mainly in Eastern Europe, where they tended to concentrate on what was observable—cleanliness, wax levels, purity, colour and so on. As we have acquired more understanding of the chemical constituents of propolis so standards have sought to identify key chemicals and elements one would expect to find in true propolis. A combination of increasing interest in the West and a radical improvement of analytical equipment has made both authentication and quality evaluation of propolis a more important and realistic goal.

An East European standard for propolis

Government standards appeared first in the former USSR and Romania, where propolis is in regular use both as a traditional medicine and in orthodox health care. A basic standard was set by *Russian Regional Standards* in 1977.[11]

Table 4: Basic standard for propolis, *Russian Regional Standards*, 1977

Extractable substances	21.93 ± 2.22%
Oxidisability value	17.08 ± 5.52%
Waxes	27.11 ± 7.68%
Polyphenols	14.66 ± 2.34%
Mechanical impurities	9.76 ± 1.81%

A Japanese standard for propolis

The market for propolis in Japan is substantial. In 1995, total sales were estimated at around £15 million. The propolis market in Japan began to really grow in the 1980s, with supplies coming initially from Brazil where a large Japanese community had grown up after the Second World War. This propolis was expensive and finished product prices in Japan are on average 5–10 times higher than those in the UK.

In 1995 the Japan Health and Nutrition Food Association—a trade association—published a standard for both raw propolis and for propolis contained in foods.

The standard focuses on the bioflavonoid content as the most important positive ingredient. Minimum flavonoid content is set at six per cent for Chinese propolis and three per cent for Brazilian propolis, and a test for total flavonoids content is described.

The standard refers to a range of substances which propolis should not contain, including lead (not more than 200 ppm), arsenic (not more than 2 ppm), bacteria (no more than $5 \times 10_4$). Raw propolis should also contain no residual agricultural chemicals, antibiotics (tetracycline), PCBs (polycholorbiphenyl), or diethylene glycol.

A UK standard for propolis

In 1995, the UK Department of Health, in the wake of the crisis over lead, effectively told UK manufacturers to solve the problem or withdraw propolis from the market. The UK Health Food Manufacturers Association (HFMA) took on the task of producing a clear unambiguous specification or standard for propolis as a whole. The purpose of the standard was to protect and inform consumers as well as to protect legitimate manufacturers from unscrupulous competition.

It took the group nearly four years to produce this specification, along with an appropriate test methodology.[12] The problem was that few were in agreement as to which of the many elements in propolis the group should be looking for. Most agreed that the bioflavonoids were important, but which ones and in what quantities?

Initially it had been thought that the bioflavonoid quercetin would be a central component to look for and measure. In the absence of any mutually recognised analytical test for propolis, it had become an accepted belief, held by many producers, that if their product had a significant proportion of quercetin in it then they could be sure it was propolis. This turned out to be a myth.

At the time, not all manufacturers were buying and refining raw propolis themselves from known sources. Many small-scale producers were buying imported extracts which claimed to be 3:1, 4:1 and, as we have seen, 5:1. Because quality controllers had decided they should be looking and testing for quercetin in their raw material, some unscrupulous producers were obliging by providing a product with high levels of quercetin added.

The group turned to the work of New Zealander Dr K Markham, who had been exploring the bioflavonoid content of propolis using HPLC (high performance liquid chromatography).

HPLC analysis can produce a 'fingerprint' for propolis by recording the way the different biochemicals in it refract light as they pass through a column in solution. Different biochemicals refract light at different points over time. Under uniform conditions, a particular biochemical will always register at the same time point. Identifying each peak is achieved by using pure samples of the biochemicals you believe to be present and matching up the peaks with the sample being analysed. The diagram below illustrates how the flavonoids reveal themselves in a typical high-performance liquid chromatogram.

Each peak in this chromatogram represents and identifies a different biochemical. Many of them are bioflavonoids. The three tallest peaks other than cinnamic acid and the standard compound used—that is peaks 3, 6 and 7—are all bioflavonoids: pinocembrin, chrysin and galangin. A number of the other peaks are biochemical variations on these flavonoids.

The UK Propolis Specification Group chose these three flavonoids as key identifiers, not necessarily actives, in propolis. If they are present in the propolis product tested in appropriate quantities, then the propolis can be said to meet specification.

A TYPICAL CHROMATOGRAM OF PROPOLIS TINCTURE RECORDED AT 200NM

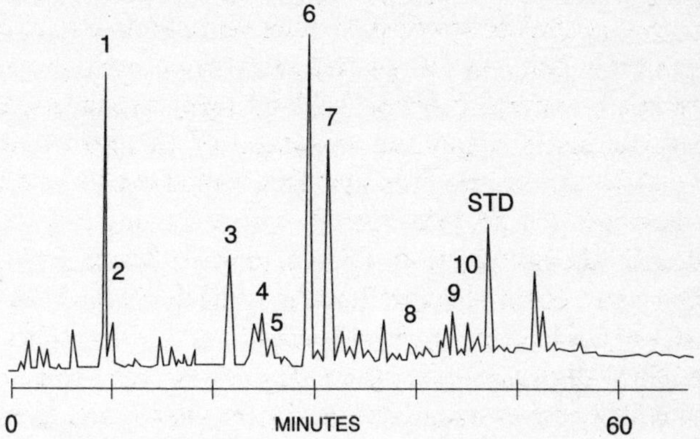

PEAK	FLAVONOID	REACTION TIME
1.	Cinnamic acid	(RT 10.51 min.)
2.	Pinobanksin	(RT 11.18 min.)
3.	Pinocembrin	(RT 24.51 min.)
4.	Pinobanksin 3-acetate	(RT 27.85 min.)
5.	1,1-dymethylallycaffeic acid	(RT 28.60 min.)
6.	Chrysin	(RT 31.33 min.)
7.	Galangin	(RT 33.65 min.)
8.	Pinocembrin 7-methyl ether	(RT 41.40 min.)
9.	Tryst 7-methyl ether	(RT 45.05 min.)
10.	Galangin 7-methyl ether	(RT 47.10 min.)
STD	**Internal Standard** 5,7-dimethyl-4'-methoxyflavanone	(RT 49.10 min.)

Working with a well-known research laboratory, the group has adapted Dr Markham's methodology to produce an easily replicable and cost-effective test for manufacturers.

Two separate specifications have been produced, one for raw propolis and a second for purified raw (refined–extracted) propolis (See appendix 1). Raw propolis must contain at least one per cent of each of the bioflavonoids, galangin, pinocembrin and chrysin. Purified raw propolis, that the 'total alcohol and or water-extracted matter obtained from raw propolis meeting the relevant standard, with addition of no further ingredient,' must contain a minimum of two per cent of each of the bioflavonoids. As can be seen from figure 1 there are more bioflavonoids than this in propolis but the UK specification has chosen to identify the three largest and seek specific quantification of them.

The UK specification for purified raw propolis includes criteria other than the presence of bioflavonoids. For example, purified raw propolis must contain less than 1 ppm lead and arsenic and not contain more than five per cent wax following extraction.

All members of the UK Health Food Manufacturers Association must attain this minimum standard, although non-members can apply for recognition that they have met the standard if they can show that their product meets the minimum requirements. Each manufacturer meeting the standard may reproduce a mark on its product which informs consumers that the particular product meets the standard.

At the moment the specification does not include any test for the biological activity of propolis—for example, does the product have antibiotic or anti-inflammatory properties? Consumers not only want to know that the product is, what it says it is, but that it does what it claims to do, in other words that it is effective. This remains a very difficult and contentious area. Consumers may want to do know what particular natural medicines are good for, yet it remains illegal for manufacturers to tell them.

PROPOLIS—FOOD OR MEDICINE?

It was Hippocrates, the founder of modern medicine, who said, 'Let food be your medicine and medicine your food'. To him and to many present-day natural therapists, food and medicine are two complementary sides of the same coin, helping you to stay well and to combat illness. However, since the advent of modern chemical medicine—synthetic chemical drugs designed to treat particular symptoms—a gulf has grown up between the two. Today, food is seen by many as fodder for the body, fuel to keep us going and to provide energy. Medicines, on the other hand, have become mysterious, complex and abstract chemical entities, designed to provide highly targeted 'fixes' for illness when it occurs. This could not be further from the truth. Today we consume many foods in the full knowledge that they have specific physiological effects; fruits for their vitamins and bioflavonoids (antioxidant effects), garlic for the heart, calcium to build bones, vegetables rich in iron for the blood and so on, but according to most Western laws this makes them medicines, which can only be sold if they have been licensed.

European law is fairly typical. According to EEC Directive 65/65 medicines are: 'Any substance or combination of substances presented for treating or preventing disease in human beings or animals' and 'Any substance or combination of substances which may be administered to human beings or animals with a view to making a diagnosis or to restoring, correcting or modifying physiological functions in human beings or animals is likewise considered a medicinal product.'

Readers will note that '*substances or combinations of substances*' have to be '*presented for treating or preventing disease*' or '*with a view to making a diagnosis or to restoring, correcting or modifying physiological functions . . .*'

What this means, in effect, is that producers and manufacturers of natural medicines (without specific medicine licences) can sell their products, providing they do not inform the public what they are for! Compare this situation to that of, say, the manufacturer of the latest tractor fitted with every conceivable new function—he may sell his tractor but he is not allowed to tell his customers what the tractor can do.

Supporters of this system argue that the public must be protected. They argue that if manufacturers of natural medicines want to make 'medical claims', i.e. that the product may alter the physiology of the body or, more specifically in the case of propolis, it may help a particular condition, asthma or arthritis for example, then they should apply for a medicine licence.

The problem is that the licensing system is designed for a radically different kind of medicine. It is designed for synthetic chemical medicines, tightly targeted to combat single disease conditions. It cannot work for natural medicines. Furthermore, it involves huge costs which can only be justified if the end product can be patented. Patenting natural medicines would be like trying to patent water.

In the past, during the time when natural medicines were not widely used, government agencies regulating medicine law would turn a blind eye to manufacturers *presenting* products as able to help with particular conditions. Oddly enough, since the renaissance of natural medicine, legislators appear to be getting tougher. In the UK legislation has recently been passed which allows regulators to look not just at what manufacturers claim directly, but to 'consider what impression of the product an *averagely well-informed consumer* would be likely to gain.' So, if an averagely well-informed consumer believed that a product would have some particular positive effect—because, for example, the product was targeted at a particular health group (people with arthritis), or because he/she had read about its use in treating a particular health problem—then they would have the power to label that product a medicine and withdraw it from the market if it did not have an 'appropriate authorization,' i.e. a medicine licence.

Virtually everyone believes that this situation is nonsense and that what is required is another category of medicines, effectively, natural medicines, somewhere in between straight foods and chemical medicines. Everyone agrees that the public needs to be protected against unscrupulous operators and that there needs to be an appropriate regulatory framework that can assure consumers that these natural products are safe and effective. Emphasis, though, is on the word 'appropriate'. Evaluating natural medicines with the standards established to evaluate chemical medicines would be like comparing the potential of unique human beings with sophisticated but nonetheless mechanical robots.

Fortunately, consumers themselves are beginning to exercise considerable influence in this field. In recent years, where government has sought to restrict the sale of some natural medicines on the grounds that they are not licensed, it has faced well-organised resistance, which has forced it to back down. Politicians now realise that consumers feel strongly on this matter and parliamentary support is growing for natural medicines to have appropriate protection. As a member of the European Community however, Britain cannot act alone and natural medicines are as yet a long way from having the protection they need.

CONSUMER INFORMATION

Providing consumers with good quality information about propolis has not been easy. As we have seen, it is illegal for manufacturers to refer to the 'medicinal' benefits of propolis, either directly or indirectly. Many have sought to circumvent the legislation by encouraging others, usually writers and researchers, to speak about propolis. In this way a patchwork of information begins to circulate which can be of variable quality. Facts which appear in newspaper or magazine articles tend to get recycled endlessly, sometimes without verification.

The Propolis Information Bureau, started in 1994, and run by the Templegarth Trust, a natural health trust based in Lincolnshire, has in the seven years of its existence handled around 60,000 enquiries about propolis. It now receives enquiries from all over the world. The Bureau publishes a series of leaflets and pamphlets about propolis, some of which have been translated into Japanese and Korean, as well as selling a range of other books and publications about propolis. It has done more than any other single organisation in the UK to get good quality information out to consumers.

Consumers, however, are still confused about which products are the best quality and the best value for money. Perhaps what the natural health industry needs, is a body similar to the Consumers' Association in the UK or the Consumers' Union in USA, prepared to undertake serious comparative research of differing brands of natural products. Such a body would be able to name both the best and the worst in the same way that the CA and the CU have been prepared to take on the manufacturers of cars, toasters and washing machines, who do not deliver what they claim. This would achieve two purposes. Firstly, it would provide good quality information and advice to consumers, and secondly, it would provide a membership base for a genuinely independent and powerful consumer voice for natural medicine users.

CHAPTER 10

Making Your Own Medicines

We have seen that when a product like propolis becomes popular, it is not always easy to identify which products are the best value for money or indeed which are the best quality. One way around this dilemma is to do what man has done for thousands of years, that is to make your own medicines. This may sound both difficult and dangerous: in fact it is neither.

First, you will need to get hold of some raw propolis with which to make your base tincture and from which you can then make all the other products. Try contacting your local beekeeper, if you know one, or else contact the British Beekeepers Association (address at the back) and they should be able to help locate one near you.

Not all beekeepers collect propolis but most should be happy to extract the small amount you will need for your test batch. If you do need to pay for the propolis, bear in mind that the current world price for raw propolis is around $15–$20 per kilo when you are buying by the ton, so you could reasonably expect to pay up to £5 for 250 grams. But don't be surprised if you are given it for free. If you are unable to get it from a beekeeper, then you could try contacting one of the principal manufacturers and refiners of propolis products. You can check to see if the propolis is still OK by using a simple test devised by some Canadian beekeepers. Put half a teaspoon of finely ground raw propolis into a small cup of fresh milk and leave in a warm temperature for four days. 'If the milk is still fresh after that time your propolis is OK.'[1]

MAKING A PROPOLIS TINCTURE

There are two ways of calculating the concentration of propolis. One way is to calculate the weight of dissolved solids in a given amount of solvent in the finished tincture. The other, simpler and more practical method recommended here is based on dissolving a known proportion of raw propolis in your chosen solvent.

Two solvents are most commonly used—alcohol and propylene glycol. Whilst alcohol provides the most effective and easiest solvent to use, extracts made from propylene glycol can be more appropriate when making some particular products, e.g. water-based creams.

To make a 25 per cent (1:4) alcohol extract you will need 250g of propolis plus four times that weight/volume in alcohol, i.e. approximately 1 litre of alcohol, depending on the strength of the alcohol.

The kind of alcohol you use is important for two reasons. Firstly, if you are going to use the end product on yourself or on your pets then *you must use food grade or drinking alcohol*. Denatured alcohol, which is much cheaper to buy, contains chemicals designed to stop it being drunk. The residues left by denatured alcohols can have adverse effects if consumed. Secondly, research has shown that you get more of the active elements out of propolis if you use 70 per cent or higher proof alcohol. You should be able to buy this grade alcohol from your local chemist. You can, however, use commercially distilled drinking alcohol—gin, rum, whisky, vodka etc. Whilst these products are not as strong and effective extractants as pure ethanol, they are perfectly adequate for home use.

Take your propolis and remove any obvious contaminants as best you can, i.e. pieces of wood etc. Cut the propolis into small pieces and place it in a large clean jar. Pour on the alcohol and close with a tight-fitting lid. You should leave the propolis soaking for a minimum of one week, shaking it regularly every day. Keep the bottle in a warm, dark place during this time. This long soak is important. Research has shown that optimum extraction takes between 7–12 days.[2] Some people find that warming the liquid helps dissolution but it is best to use as little heat as possible as this can damage the bioflavonoids. Remember, though, that alcohol is a highly inflammable liquid and should not be placed anywhere near a direct flame.

The resulting liquid is first filtered through a fine cloth or through paper filters. Muslin is ideal or coffee filters can be used. Following this first filtration, place the filtered product in the fridge for a day or so and then filter again, using as fine a filter as possible. Store the liquid in clean dark-coloured bottles if possible and store away from direct sunlight. Propolis tincture made in this way will last indefinitely. Propolis is, in any case, bactericidal but alcohol over 30 per cent concentration is also an effective preservative.

The method is exactly the same when using propylene glycol but it is probably better to use only 10 per cent raw propolis, i.e. 100g to a litre of glycol, as glycol is not as effective a solvent as alcohol. You may also need to use a little heat to help the propolis dissolve if using glycol.

USING THE TINCTURE

We have seen how you can use alcoholic tinctures for a variety of purposes. Take a few drops a day to stay well, to boost your immune system or prevent coughs and colds. It is best to put the drops in warm liquid—juice or tea—as the resin in the tincture tends to stick to the container. You can also mix the tincture with honey or place a few drops on bread.

The tincture can be used to treat cuts, grazes, burns, dermatitis, wounds and infections.[3] Less than one per cent of people are allergic to propolis so remember to apply small amounts to the affected area to start with and discontinue if a significant allergic reaction is observed. The resinous part of the tincture forms a membrane over wounds, avoiding the need for a dressing. As we have seen, it assists the regeneration of tissue, and reduces bleeding and pain.

Propylene glycol tinctures can be used in the same way. Indeed, external use on wounds and burns may be more appropriate because the liquid does not sting as much as the alcohol-based product. Bear in mind, though, that it is not advisable for humans to consume more than 1.5g of glycol per day[4] so if you are taking the tincture internally on a regular basis, it is probably better to use one that is alcohol-based.

PROPOLIS SPRAYS

Both alcohol and propylene glycol propolis solutions can be mixed with appropriate alcoholic herbal extracts to produce a spray suitable for treatment of mouth and nasal problems. A five per cent extract of either propolis solution is mixed with 1:20 extract of regalis, anis, eucalyptus or mint, according to taste. The solution can be further diluted and bottled in a small mechanical spray. The solution is sprayed on the affected areas and has been found to be effective in treating mouth ulcers and nasal congestion as well as for treating halitosis (bad breath) If you prefer, you can use a propolis solution on its own. Glycol solutions are sometimes preferred for this use as the liquid does not evaporate as quickly as the alcohol solutions and does not sting as much when applied to sore and affected areas.

The spray has also been found to be a useful way of delivering propolis to burns, wounds and skin infections as it delivers a fine film of propolis to the affected area without the potential for further damage. Propylene glycol solutions are again preferred for the same reasons mentioned above.

PROPOLMEL

This recipe, developed by Jacob Kaal,[5] has been used principally to stimulate the glands and as a preventative against infection and inflammations of the stomach and intestine as well as for the treatment of prostate conditions.

One part of 25 per cent propolis extract weight (produced as above) is mixed with seven parts honey and two parts fresh pollen where available. According to Kaal, the pollen tends to raise blood pressure whilst the honey restores the balance. You may wish to experiment with different proportions of honey, propolis and pollen. Mix the propolis and pollen with a small amount of honey before integrating it with the balance of honey.

Using the propolmel as a base you can also add other bee

products and herbs designed to achieve specific effects. For example, add royal jelly and a dash of ginseng and lotus extract to produce a nourishing and invigorating tonic for older people suffering from chronic illness or convalescence following illness or an operations.[6]

PROPOLIS AND HONEY

Adding propolis to honey is an excellent way of masking the taste of propolis and combining the complementary function of honey and propolis. It is also an excellent way of getting children to take propolis. Products of this kind should be stored in dark jars in a cool place.

A mixture of honey and propolis has been used to treat burns successfully. The burned area is covered in honey and propolis, bandaged and left for a number of days.

PROPOLIS VASELINE OINTMENT

For this ointment you will need to evaporate the alcohol or glycol from the tincture to produce a concentrated extract. You can do this by gently warming the tincture in a water bath until the liquid is reduced to a sticky consistency. You will not be able to get the liquid down to a dry powder. Slowly mix the thick reduced extract with Vaseline in the ratio of one part propolis extract to 20 parts of Vaseline if using the alcohol extract, and one part to 10 if using the glycol extract. Again, a little heat applied via a water bath may be useful here. Mix well by hand or with an ordinary electric mixer until the ointment takes on a uniform and darker colour.

You can use this ointment externally, with the same provisos as mentioned above, to treat ulcers and burns in humans, and abscesses and festering wounds in animals. Where a wound is open, it is advisable to apply the ointment around the outside of the wound first. This encourages the tissue to heal progressively towards the centre of the affected area over time. Continue to apply until the wound is completely healed.

PROPOLIS OIL-BASED OINTMENT

For this ointment use two parts by weight of the propolis extract produced in the method above to one part beeswax, seven parts lanolin and 10 parts butter of palm, cacao or similar.

First, melt the beeswax in a water bath, slowly stirring in the lanolin. When the mixture has cooled, blend in the pre-mixed butter and propolis to produce a homogenous mixture. This soothing ointment can be used for a variety of skin problems by being gently massaged into the affected areas.

PROPOLIS CREAM

Rather than make your own, you can add propolis to most base creams. You may need to experiment a little to find the right proportions—usually somewhere between one–five per cent. Most creams are water-based and therefore you may find that the propylene glycol solution mixes more effectively with the cream.

Jacob Kaal[7] tells us that the 'contractile strength of propolis combats the formation of wrinkles on the face and causes liver spots to disappear.' Most base creams, whether they be designed as moisturising, rejuvenating or curative, can be improved with the additions of relatively small proportions (one–two per cent by weight) of propolis. In particular, these fortified creams can be useful in treating fungal diseases of the skin as well as psoriasis, particularly when taken in conjunction with propolis internally. Patients who find stronger propolis ointments irritating because of an allergic response can often benefit from using the milder creams.

PROPOLIS FACIAL MASKS

Dr Murat[8] tells us of a patient whose face 'was so seriously wrinkled that it looked like a sponge.' Apparently, after a few months of propolis facial mask left on overnight, 'she looked twenty years younger and her face had a lovely youthful appearance.' Sonowski[9] devised the following recipe for a propolis facial mask. Five parts filler (this can be fuller's earth, china clay, kaolin, bentonite or a mixture of all of them), four parts 50 per cent glycerol solution, five parts 50 per cent propolis solution, and an appropriate amount of perfume or essential oils. The propolis extract is mixed with the glycerol. This mixture is then mixed with the filler and the perfume. This recipe may be varied with the addition of other appropriate herbal mixtures with a reputation for cleansing. The mixture is then applied thickly to the face and left on overnight.

Krochmal[10] has a slightly simpler recipe for a cleansing mask for oily skins. This mask should not be mixed until immediately prior to use, as it does not contain a preservative and would otherwise deteriorate quickly. The ingredients are in parts per volume: four parts fuller's earth (or similar product), one part rose water, one part lemon juice, two parts honey, one part 5–10 per cent propolis extract, either in ethanol or glycol. Whether in ethanol or glycol the propolis solution should be diluted, enabling water to be added more easily. Prepare the rose water by adding a few drops of the essential oil to water or by preparing an infusion of rose petals. Once again, this recipe can be varied by the additions of differing appropriate herbal tinctures or essential oils, and once more the mixture is spread over the whole face and left to carry out its work for a number of hours, preferably overnight.

PROPOLIS MASSAGE OIL

To produce a propolis massage oil, Felix Murat[11] suggests mixing one part propolis extract with two parts of a base oil (this may be sunflower, sesame, grape seed, olive or sweet almond oil) and 20 parts of any traditional massage oil. This produces a regenerative and invigorating effect when massaged into the skin.

PROPOLIS TABLETS

Again the recipe is in parts by weight. You will need one part gum arabic, one part water, one part propolis extract (ideally reduced from propylene glycol) and 10 parts powdered sugar, pollen or wholewheat flour, and flavouring if required.

First, mix the water with the gum arabic until it forms a homogenous mass. Then slowly stir in the propolis extract and the pollen, sugar or flour. You may have to experiment a little with this recipe.

What you are aiming for is a well-mixed but stiff consistency, which you can roll into a ball-like pastry. Then spread a surface with powdered sugar and roll out a thin layer. You can then cut this propolis 'pastry' into small squares or circles, placing them on a sugared board to dry and go hard. You can finish them off in a low oven if you prefer.

The resulting tablets may not look too much like today's professionally-made tablets but they will work just as well. You can use them like lozenges after dental treatment or if you have mouth ulcers, by allowing them to slowly dissolve in your mouth.

PROPOLIS TOOTHPASTE AND MOUTHWASH

A number of commercial propolis toothpastes are now available on the market. They often have a very low proportion of propolis in them. They are used to help maintain everyday oral hygiene and prevent dental decay via the antibiotic anti-plaque properties of propolis. Rather than make your own toothpaste, from start to finish, it is probably easier to buy natural toothpaste, already on the market and mix in extra propolis. You can do this by undoing the folded end of the tube, pushing out the paste and mixing it with one–five per cent by weight of the propolis extract you are left with after you have evaporated either the glycol or ethanol liquid.

A simple mouthwash can also be produced by adding 10–15 drops of propolis liquid to a glass of warm water and using it to rinse the mouth instead of using a chemical preparation. Unlike traditional mouthwashes you can finish off by swallowing it and getting the added benefit of the propolis internally.

ANAESTHETIC PROPOLIS PASTE

Propolis has gained a substantial reputation for treating dental problems, including mouth ulcers, gingyvitis, and pericorinitis. As well as addressing the inflammatory nature of these conditions, propolis also acts as an anaesthetic, reducing pain in the mouth.

The following recipe has been designed to bring out the anaesthetic properties of propolis.[12] The ingredients (in parts by weight) are 10 parts lanolin, 10 parts unbleached beeswax, 10 parts petrolatum (Vaseline), two parts ethyl aminobenzoate, three parts clove oil and 15 parts propolis (50 per cent concentration ethanol extract).

Melt the beeswax and the Vaseline in a water bath and, as the mixture begins to cool, stir in the lanolin. When the mixture has cooled to around 40°C (104°F) then add the propolis and the other ingredients.

Apply the paste to the affected area and encourage the patient to try and keep it there. Alternatively, if you can find some clean, raw propolis, chew it until it has the consistency of chewing gum and mould it round the affected tooth or area if possible.

PROPOLIS SUNTAN LOTIONS

Add between two–five per cent by weight of reduced propylene glycol extract to your chosen suntan solution. In this way you can add the tissue-regenerating properties of propolis to the sun-blocking effect of the lotion. Dr Murat[13] confirms that propolis 'acts as a screen against the ultra-violet rays of the sun and prevents sunburn and sores.'

Apply first to a small area to be sure that you are not one of the few people who have an allergic skin reaction.

PROPOLIS HAIR PREPARATIONS

In the manufacturers' survey of propolis users mentioned earlier, a number of people referred to the improved quality and texture of their hair as a result of taking propolis. Dr Murat[14] tells us that massaging propolis oil into the hair 'makes the hair more natural-looking.' He also tells us that it 'stops itching and often eliminates dandruff.'

You can make your own anti-dandruff lotion in the following way.[15] The ingredients you will need (in parts by weight) are: one part of 10 per cent ethanol propolis solution (made as above), five parts laurylsulphate, 37 parts 100 per cent ethanol, 57 parts rain water or boiled water.

First, mix the one part propolis with the 37 parts ethanol and then mix the five parts laurylsulphate with 57 parts of boiled or rain water. Finally, mix the two solutions together. Use like a shampoo, leaving on the hair for five minutes before rinsing.

You can make a conventional shampoo by adding around one–two per cent parts by weight to a shampoo base of your own choice. Depending on what is in the shampoo you use, some may lose their viscosity when mixed with alcohol. Also, take care not to put too much propolis extract in the shampoo because propolis can stain the skin.

Afterword

'From around 2002 onwards people will get a sore throat on Tuesday and be dead by Friday.' This is the apocalyptic vision of George Poste, former Director of Research at the pharmaceutical company Smith Kline Beecham. He believes that we have run out of time to develop the new breed of antibiotics we need to destroy the ever-growing number of highly sophisticated bacteria now resistant to our most powerful antibiotics. Poste believes that even if we survive this wave of resistant bacteria, 'The next wave will come in 2020 to 2025. It is an absolutely predictable outcome.'

Whilst not everyone shares this bleak analysis, many leading doctors and scientists are extremely concerned about the increasing number of antibiotic-resistant bacteria, such as:

- *Methicillin-Resistant Staphylococcus aureus* (MRSA) which is most commonly found in infectious wounds, the skin and the bloodstream and is present in over 60 per cent of UK hospitals.
- *Penicillin-Resistant Streptococcus pneumonia* which is common in problems like child ear infections, pneumonia and meningitis.
- *Multi-Resistant Neisseria gonorrhoeae*, which causes the venereal disease gonorrhoea.
- *Multi-Drug-Resistant Tuberculosis* (MDRTB). It was thought that tuberculosis had been cured. It is, however, making a serious comeback in the UK and now very difficult to treat.
- *Vanomycin Resistant Enterococcus* (VRE), which infects wounds, the urinary tract and causes heart valve infections. Mainly found in hospitals.

Bacterial resistance, however, is not a new problem. It turns out that *Staphylococcus aureus*, the most common problem bacterium, took just 18 months, following the first introduction of penicillin, to discover a way of chopping it up and neutralising it. By the end of the 1950s, 90 per cent of all the *Staphylococcus aureus* strains had become resistant. It took the infinitely ingenious *Staphylococcus aureus* a mere further 18 months to crack the code of Methicillin, the new antibiotic developed to overcome this resistance, following its introduction in 1959. Notwithstanding this, in the early 1960s the US Surgeon General announced that infectious disease had been conquered!

As Professor Gary French, head of microbiology at St Thomas's Hospital, London, says, 'Humans are not so bright. They think about things, but bugs only think about one thing: surviving.' Whilst antibiotics and other synthetic drugs have saved millions of lives, there has clearly been a huge and, until recently, hidden and devastating price to pay. In our over-use of antibiotics we have created a race of superbugs. The enemy, far from being conquered, has become stronger.

However, medical researchers are beginning to question their search for the Holy Grail of single active ingredients. Some are starting to realise that some of the answers might be back where medicine started, i.e. with the whole plant, not with just one single part of it. They are beginning to realise that the biochemical packages contained in plants work as a team, synergistically. Of course, some particular biochemicals may have a key role to play in achieving a particular pharmacological function, like an entrepreneurial leader in a business, but without the rest of the team the job will not get done.

In propolis, we found that the flavonoids in general and perhaps the caffeic acid derivatives in particular, are important in achieving the wide range of pharmacological effects it is credited with. However, attempts to isolate these products have not on the whole been successful and research refers again and again to the greater effectiveness of the whole product.

The big question for modern medicine, however, is whether natural products like propolis can really help us to avoid the crisis of modern antibiotics spelt out by Poste. The incredible body and range of research about propolis that we have covered in this short book would seem to answer yes.

Two pieces of research in particular point the way to a future role for propolis. Firstly, the pioneering work of Grange and Davey in 1990 at the UK Heart and Lung Institute, in London. They found that propolis was capable of destroying MRSA (*Methicillin Resistant Staphylococcus aureus*). It seems that where a bacterium is faced with the whole exponentially-complex biochemical package of a natural antibiotic, it cannot decode it and evolve around it in the same way as it can with a single synthetic compound.

Secondly, the work carried out at the Kazan Veterinary Institute in 1973 showed that mixing propolis with an antibiotic can improve the effectiveness of the antibiotic by between 10 and 100 times. If this is true and can be shown to work in clinical trials then the benefits could be enormous. Not only could we radically reduce our intake of antibiotics but it is possible that propolis could reduce other side effects of antibiotics. The production of Propocillin (a combination of propolis and antibiotics) could potentially help fight disease and save millions of pounds on health care.

Propolis though is not just an antibiotic. We have seen that it has anti-inflammatory, anti-fungal, anti-cancer and even anaesthetic properties. It is a different kind of medicine. Synthetic antibiotics work by destroying bacteria, propolis appears to work by disarming them. Whilst it is used by many to fight disease, another of its major strengths lies in preventing disease. Research into the use of propolis in preventing and treating flu showed that its most effective role was as a prophylactic, preventing one from getting the disease, rather than curing one of it. Again this is an important distinction between natural medicines like propolis and synthetic drug-based medicines. Their primary role is to help one's own system fight disease rather than defeat one particular group of bacteria or viruses. Propolis is never going to operate like Vancomycin or Methicillin but then neither is it going to create the same long-term problems.

Only now are we beginning to realise that natural medicines are infinitely more complex than synthetic drugs—propolis—is perhaps one of the most complex. Despite the mass of research conducted into propolis, we still have much to learn about its properties and potential. A recent piece in a British national newspaper described how a group of nuns were using propolis to successfully treat Alzheimer's disease, a growing health problem nowadays. If this is true and not just the so-called placebo effect, then how is it working and how can it be used to best treat patients? Recent research into the treatment of Alzheimer's disease has suggested that improved increase in the blood flow to the brain can help. We have seen earlier that propolis can act to dilate blood vessels, so perhaps this is why it appears to be helping with Alzheimer's. But until we get further serious research into propolis we are not going to know.

It is said that necessity is the mother of invention. Perhaps, in the case of propolis, necessity will be the mother of reinvention as the deepening crisis encourages us revisit the medicines of the past with all the real benefits of the science of today.

Useful Addresses

International Bee Research Association, 18 North Road, Cardiff, CF10 3DT, UK.
Tel: +44(0)29 20 372409 Fax: +44(0)29 20 665522
E-mail: ibra@cf.ac.uk
www.cf.ac.uk/ibra/

American Apitherapy Society
www.apitherapy.com

British Beekeepers Association, National Beekeeping Centre, National Agricultural Centre, Stoneleigh Park, Warwickshire, CV8 2LG, UK.
www.bbka.org.uk

Bees for Development, Troy, Monmouth, NP5 4AB, UK.
www.planbee.org.uk
E-mail busy@planbee.org.uk

Propolis Information Bureau, PO Box 6, Louth, Lincolnshire, LN11 8XL.

Apimondia, International Federation of Beekeepers' Association
www.becheeping.com/apimondia
E-mail Apimondia@mclink.it

BeeNet UK
SteveTurner@amigabee.or.uk

Central Science Laboratory, National Bee Unit UK, Sand Hutton, York, YO41 1LZ, UK.
Tel: 01904 462000
Fax: 01904 462111
E-mail mbew@csl.gov.uk

Rothamsted Experimental Station, IACR Rothamstead
Harpenden, Hertfordshire. A15 2JQ, UK.
Tel: +44(0)1582 763133
Fax: +44(0)1582 760981
www.iacr.bbsrc.ac.uk
Email: res.helpdesk@bbsrc.ac.uk

Propolis-Producing Companies

Natural Laboratories, 7 East Court Mews, Charlton Kings, Cheltenham, Gloucestershire, UK.
Power Health, Pocklington, North Yorkshire, UK.
Bee Health, East Ayton, Scarborough, North Yorkshire, UK.
CC Pollen, Phoenix, Arizona, USA.
Beehive Botanicals, Hayward, Wisconsin, USA.

References

Introduction Propolis—Defender of the City

1 Steiner, R (1923). *Nine Lectures on Bees*, Rudolf Steiner Press.
2 Dr George Jacoby, quoted in Garret, (1994). *The Coming Plague: Newly Emerging Diseases in a World Out of Balance*, Penguin.
3 Dr Harold Neu, *ibid.*
4 Garret, L (1994). *The Coming Plague: Newly Emerging Diseases in a World Out of Balance*, Penguin.

Chapter 1 What is Propolis

1 Kustenmacher, cited in Cizmarik, J., Macicka, M. and Matel, I. (1978). *Analysis and considerations on theories concerning production of propolis*, Apimondia Publishing House.
2 Rosch, *ibid.*
3 Phillip, *ibid.*
4 Cizmarik, J., Macicka, M. and Matel, I. (1978) *Analysis and considerations on theories concerning production of propolis*, Apimondia Publishing House.
5 Cuellar, A., Rojas Hernandez, N. M., Martinez Perez, J. (1990). New antimicrobial structure from propolis collected in Cuba, *Revista Cubana de Farmacia* 24(1): 51–8.
6 Greenaway, W., Scaysbrook, T., Whatley, F. R. (1990). The composition and plant origins of propolis. A report of work at Oxford, *Bee World*, 71(3): 107–18.
7 Frederich, T. (1999). Occasional Paper, Apimondia Publishing House.
8 Greenaway (1990).
9 Petri, G., Lemberkovics, E., Foldvari, M. (1988) Examination of differences between propolis (bee glue) produced from

different floral environments. In Lawrence, B., Mookherjee, B. D., Willis, B. J., Elsevier—Science Publishers 439–46.
10 Gabrys, J., Konechi, Z., Krol, W., Scheller, S., Shani, (eds), (1988). J. (1986) *Flavours and Fragrances*, product (propolis) as identified and quantified by gas-liquid chromatography, *Pharmacol. 180* Res.—Communications 18(6): 513–8.
11 Murat, F. (1982). *Propolis—The Eternal Natural Healer*, Privately published.

Chapter 2 The Role of Propolis in the Hive

1 Ransome, H. (1986). *The Sacred Bee*, Bee Books New and Old.
2 Ainiri, A., *ibid.*
3 Murat, F. (1982). *Propolis—The Eternal Natural Healer*, privately published.
4 Leipus, *ibid.*
5 Ghisalberti, E. L. (1979). Propolis: A review. *Bee World*, 60(2): 59–84.
6 Mlagan, V., Sulimanovic, D. (1982). Action of propolis solutions on *Bacillus larvae*, *Apiacta*, (17): 16–20.
7 Meresta, T. and Meresta, L. (1988). Sensitivity of *Bacillus larvae* to an extract of propolis *in vitro*. *Medycyna Weterynaryjna*, 44(3): 169–70.

Chapter 3 The Folk History and Use of Propolis

1 Kahun Papyri, quoted in Ransome, H. (1986). *The Sacred Bee*, Bee Books New and Old.
2 Budge, E. Wallis. (1901). *Egyptian Magic*, cited in Ransome, H. (1986). *The Sacred Bee*, Bee Books New and Old.
3 Nizami's *Alexander's Exploits*, cited in Ransome, H. (1986). *The Sacred Bee*, Bee Books New and Old.
4 King, L. W. (1903). *Babylonian Religion and Mythologies*, cited in Ransome, H. (1986). *The Sacred Bee*, Bee Books New and Old.
5 Budge, E. Wallis (ed.) (1896). *Life and Exploits of Alexander*, C. J. Clay & Sons.

6 Budge, E. Wallis (ed.). *Syriac Book of Medicine*, cited in Ransome, H. (1986). *The Sacred Bee*, Bee Books New and Old.
7 Ransome, H. (1986). *The Sacred Bee*, Bee Books New and Old.
8 Murat, F. (1982). *Propolis—The Eternal Natural Healer*, privately published.
9 Pliny. *Natural History*, cited in Ransome, H. (1986). *The Sacred Bee*, Bee Books New and Old.
10 Dioscorides, cited in Hill, R. (1977). *Propolis—Natural Antibiotic*, Thorson Press.
11 Celsus, *ibid.*
12 The Koran (Sura XVI)—The Bee.
13 Avicenna, quoted in Makashvii, Z. A. (1978). *The History of Propolis*, Apimondia Publishing House.
14 Gerard, J. (1597). *The Historie of Plants*.
15 Culpeper, N. (1653). *Complete Herbal*.
16 Green, T. (1824). *The Universal Herbal*, Caxton Press.
17 *ibid.*
18 Makashvii, Z. A. (1978). *The History of Propolis*, Apimondia Publishing House.
19 *ibid.*
20 *ibid*
21 *ibid*
22 Nikolaev, A. B. (1978). *Defending the Bee Town*, Apimondia Publishing House.

Chapter 4 Propolis in Modern Times

1 Mansfield, P. (1994). *New Medicine for Old*, Good Health Keeping.
2 *ibid.*
3 Vosnack, M. (1978). *The Miracle of Propolis*, Thorson Publishers.
4 *ibid.*
5 Aagard, K. L. (1974). *The Natural Product Propolis—the Way to Health*, Mentor Verlag.
6 *ibid.*
7 *ibid.*

8 *ibid.*
9 Cited in *American Chiropractor* January–February 1980.
10 *ibid.*
11 Personal communication with Linda Graham of Beehive Botanicals, Wisconsin.
12 Brown, R. (1993). *The World's Only Perfect Food*, Holm Press.
13 Hill, R. (1977). *Propolis—The Natural Antibiotic*, Thorson's.
14 Murat, F. (1982). *Propolis—The Eternal Natural Healer*, Privately published.
15 Kaal, J. (1987). *Natural Medicines from Honeybees*, Kaal's Printing House.
16 Diamond, J. (1978). *BK Behavioural Kinesiology*, Harper and Row, New York.
17 Weightman, P. W. H., Garcia, C. (1997). University of Newcastle upon Tyne (awaiting publication).

Chapter 5 How does propolis work?

1 Steiner, R. (1923). *Nine Lectures on Bees*, Rudolf Steiner Press.
2 Mansfield, P. (1994). *New Medicine for Old*, Good Health Keeping.
3 Houghton, P. *Propolis as a medicine*—are there scientific reasons for its reputation? cited in Munn, P. (ed), (1998). *Beeswax and Propolis for pleasure and profit*, International Bee Research Association.
4 Mirzoeva, O. K., Sud'ina, G. F., Pushkareva, M. A., Korshunova, G. A., Sumbatyan, N. V., Varfolomeev, S. D. (1995). *Lipophilic Derivatives of Caffeic Acid as Lipoxygenase Inhibitors with Antioxidant Properties, Russian Journal of Bioorganic Chemistry*, 21(2) 124–131.
5 Airola, P. (1974). *How to Get Well*, Health Plus Publishers.
6 Havsteen B., cited in Wade, C. (1983). *Propolis: Nature's Energizer. Miracle healer from the beehive*, Keats Publishing, Inc.
7 *ibid.*
8 *ibid.*
9 Prokopovich, N. N. (1957). Propolis, a new anaesthetic (Russian), *Vrach, Delo*, 10: 1077–80.

10 Tsakov, Ts. (1973). Anaesthetic properties of propolis (Bulgarian), *Farmatsiya*, 23(2): 38–41.
11 Tsakov, Ts. (1975). Study on the locally anaesthetic properties of propolis in operations on sheep and dogs, *Propolis*, Apimondia Publishing House.
12 Paintz, M., Metzner, J. (1979). Local anaesthetic effects of propolis and some of its constituents, *Pharmazie*, December, 34 (12): 839–41.
13 Havsteen, B., cited in Wade, C. (1983). *Propolis: Nature's Energizer. Miracle healer from the beehive*, Keats Publishing, Inc.
14 Ushkalova, V. N., Murykhnich, T. P. (1973). Antacid properties of propolis (Russian), *Pcelovodstvo*, 93(12): 15–16.
15 International Bee Research Association, Cardiff, UK.
16 Feuereisl and Kraus. (1958), cited in Lavie, P., (1978). *The Antibiotic from Propolis*, Apimondia Publishing House.
17 Lavie, P. (1960). *Annals Abeille*, 3: 103–201.
18 Villannueva, V. R. *et al.* (1964). *Annales de L'Institut Pasteur* 106: 262.
19 Kivalkina, V. P., Gorshunova, V. I. (1973). The possibility to use propolis combined with antibiotics (abstract), *Antibiotiki* (Moscow), 18(3): 261–3.
20 Scheller, S., Tustanowski, J., Jurylo, B., Paradowski, Z., Obuszko, Z. (1977). Biological properties and clinical application of propolis. III. Investigation of the sensitivity of Staphylococci isolated from pathological cases to ethanol extract of propolis (EEP). Attempts on inducing resistance in laboratory Staphylococcus strain to EEP. . . . *Arzneimittelforschung*, 27(7): 1395.
21 Aspoey, E. (1977). Selective effect of propolis in the isolation of Listeria monocytogenes, *Nordisk Veteerinaermedicin*, 29(10); 440–5.
22 Metzner, J., Bekemeier, H., Paintz, M., Schneidewind, E. (1979). Antimicrobial activity of propolis and its constituents, *Pharmazie*, 34(2): 97–102.
23 Shub, T. A., Kagramanova, K. A., Voropaeva, S. D., Kivman, B. Ya. (1981). Effect of propolis on strains of Staphylococcus aureus resistant to antibiotics, *Antibiotiki*, 26(4): 268–271.

24 Pepeljnjack, S., Jalseniak, J., Maysinger, D. (1985). Flavonoid content in propolis extracts and growth inhibition of Bacillus subtilis (Yugoslavia), *Pharmazie*, 40(2): 122–3.

25 Kedzia, B., Holderna, E. (1986). Investigations on the combined action of antibiotics and propolis on Staphylococcus aureus, *Herba Palonica* 32(3/4): 187–195.

26 Simuth, J., Trnovsky, J., Jelokova, J. (1986). Inhibition of bacterial DNA-dependant RNA polymerases and restriction endonuclease by UV-absorbing components from propolis (Slovakia). *Pharmazie*, 41(2): 131–2.

27 Lindenfelser, Lloyd A. (1967). Anti-microbial activity of propolis, *American Bee Journal*, 107(3): 90–92.

28 Scheller, S., Gazda, G. (1988). The ability of ethanol extract of propolis to stimulate plaque formation in immunised mouse spleen cells, *Pharmacol. -Res. -Commun.*, 20(4): 323–28.

29 Rosenthal, C., Tamarin, R., Samish, S., Elad, Da. (1989). Demonstration of the inhibitory effect of propolis on microbial straines (abstract), XXXth International Congress of Apiculture, 557.

30 Grange, J. M., Davey, R. W. (1990). Anti-bacterial properties of propolis, *Journal of the Royal Society of Medicine*, 83: 160–1.

31 Dobrowolski, J. W., Vohora, S. B., Sharma, K., Shah, S. A., Naavi, S. A. H., Dandiya, P. C. (1991). Anti-bacterial, anti-fungal, anti-ameobic, anti-inflammatory and anti-pyretic studies on bee propolis products, *Ethnopharmacology*, 5(1): 77–82.

32 Tosi, B., Donini, A., Bamognolic, C., Bruni, A. (1996). Anti-microbial activity of some commercial extractes of propolis prepared with different solvents, *Phytotherapy Research*, 10: 335–6.

33 Mirzoeva, O. K., Grishanin, R. N., Calder, P. C. (1997). Anti-microbial action of propolis and some of its components: The effect on growth membrane potential and motility of bacteria, *Microbial -Res*, 152: 239–246.

34 Vechet, L. (1978). Effect of propolis on some species of micro-organisms and moulds, *Propolis*, Apimondia Publishing House.

35 Cizmarik, J., Trupl, J. (1975). Effects of propolis on yeasts, *Pharmazie*, 30(6): 406–407.

36 Cizmarik, J., Trupl, J. (1976). Effects of propolis on skin, *Pharmazie*, 31(1): 35.

37 Starzyk, J., Scheller, S., Szatlarski, J., Moskwa, N., Stojko, A. (1977). Biological properties and clinical application of propolis. II. Studies on the anti-protozoan activity of ethanol extract of propolis, *Arzneimittel—Forschung*, 27(6): 1198–9.

38 Metzner, J., Schneidewind, E. M. (1978). Effect of pinocembrin on the course of experimental candida infections in mice, *Mykosen*, 21(8): 257–62.

39 Pepeljnjak, S, (1982). Inhibition of growth and biosynthesis of achratoxin A in Aspergillus sulphureus NRRL 4077 by propolis extract, *Pharmazie*, 37(6): 439–40.

40 Holderna, E., Kedzia, B., (1987). Investigations upon the combined action of propolis and anti-mycotic drugs on Candida albicans, *Herba Polinica*, 33(2):145–51.

41 Valdes Gonzales, G., Rojas Hernandez, N. M., Morales, V. C. (1987). Preliminary test of the action of propolis extract on Candida albicans, (abstract), XXXIst International Congress of Apiculture, 549.

42 Millet-Clerc, J., Michel, D., Simeray, J., Chaumont, J. P. (1987). Preliminary study of the anti-fungal properties of propolis compared with some commercial products, *Plantes Medicinales et Phytotherapie* 21(1): 3–7.

43 Milena, L., Leifertova, I, Baloun, I. (1989). Fungistatic effects of propolis, *Folia Pharm. Univ.* Carol 13; 29–44.

44 Havsteen, B., cited in Wade, C. (1983). *Propolis: Nature's energizer. Miracle healer from the beehive*, Keats Publishing, Inc.

45 Oita, N., Filipovici, C., Koropitzer, R. Anti-inflammatory and antiseptic hydrophilic gel. Romanian Patent (66,963).

46 Mihail, N., Giurgea, R., Coprean, D., Popescu, H., Polinicencu G. (1984). Some data on the anti-inflammatory action of standardized propolis extract, *Revue Roumaine de Biologie*, Biologie Annals, 29(2): 129–32.

47 Papay, V., Toth, L., Soltesz, M., Nagy, E., Litkei, Gy., Dinya, Z., Gabor, M., Szallai, J., (1986). The pharmacological activities of the fractions and the compounds isolated from Hungarian propolis and Populi Gemma XXXth. International Congress of Apiculture, 453–56.

48 Krol, W., Scheller, S., Czuba, Z., Matsuno, J., Zydowicz, G., Shani, J., Mos, M. (1996). Inhibition of neutrophils, chemiluminescence by ethanol extract of propolis (EEP) and its phenolic compounds, *Journ. Ethnopharmacology*, 1996: 19–25.

49 Mirzoeva, O. K., Calder, P. C. (1996). The effect of propolis and its components on eiconsanoid production during the inflammatory response, *Prostaglandins Leukot., Essent. Fatty Acids*, 55(6): 441–49.

50 Scheller, S., Gazda, G., Krol, W., Czuba, Z., Zajusz, A., Gabrys, J., Shani, J. (1989). The ability of ethanolic extract of propolis (EEP) to protect mice against gamma irradiation, *Zeitshrift fur Naturforschung(C)*, 44(11–12): 1049–52.

51 Berngard, K. E. (1976). Preparation of aqueous propolis solutions for treating fish and determination of its concentration in solution, *Ryb. Khoz.* (Moscow), 12: 66–67.

52 Dessouk, T. M., El- Dashlouty, A. A., El-Ebzary, M. M., Heika, H. A. (1980). Propolis and some other natural antioxidants for fats of frozen meat, *Agricultural Research Review*, 58(3): 311–321.

53 Popeskovic, D., Kepcija, D., Dimitrijevic, M., Stojanovic, N. (1980). The antioxidative properties of propolis and some of its components, *Acta Veterinaria*, 30(3/4): 133–6.

54 Kepcija, D., Dimitrijevic, M., Stojanovic, N. (1981). An investigation of the antioxidative properties of propolis, *Acta Veterinaria*, 341(4): 181–84.

55 Popovic, S., Dimitrijevic, M. (1982). The use of propolis in preservation of anatomic preparations *Acta Veterinaria*, 32(4): 227–30.

56 Yahishnlieva, N., Marinova, B., Bankova, V., Popov, S., Marekov, N. (1984). Does the antioxidant properties of propolis depend on the flavonoids present? *Institute Superieur de l'industrie alimentaire*, 31 March–4 Juin, 481–6.

57 Nishina, A. (1991). Japanese Patent. Food antioxidant preparations containing propolis.

58 Mizunu, M. (1989). Japanese Patent No. JP 01 243 794. Food packaging materials containing propolis as a preservative.

59 Okenenko, L. B. (1986). Propolis as an inhibitor of free radical lipid oxidation in salmonellosis, *Vopr. Med. Khim*, 32(3): 45–8.

60 Okonenko, L. B. (1988). Vitamin E and propolis as antioxidants after excessive administration of polyunsaturated fatty acid, *Vopr-Pitan*, (4): 68–70.

61 Krol, W., Czuba, Z., Scheller, S., Gabry, J., Grabeic, S., Shani, J. (1990). Antioxidant properties of ethanolic extract of propolis (EEP) as evaluated by inhibiting the chemiluminescence oxidation of luminol, *Biochemistry International*, 21(4): 593–7.

62 Clinescu, R., Radu, D., Militaru, M., Gdioiu, T. (1991). Antioxidant and anti-inflammatory action of propolis, *Studi si Cercetar de Biochemie*, 34(1–2): 19–25.

63 Pascual, C., Gonzalez, R., Torricella, R. G. (1994). Scavenging action of propolis extract against oxygen radicals. *Journ Ethnopharmacology*, 41: 9–13.

64 Volper, R. (1993). Biochemical activities of propolis extracts. I Standardisation and antioxidative properties of ethanolic and aqueus derivatives, *Z. Naturforschung (C)*, 48(11–12): 851–7.

65 Mackevicius, L., Cerniauskiene, L. R. (1997). Antioxidant and pro-oxidant action of propolis, XXXVth International Congress of Apiculture.

66 Mirzoeva, O. K., Sud'ina, G. F., Pushkareva, M. A., Korshunova, G. A., Sumbatyan, N. V., Varfolomeev, S. D. (1994). Lipophilic derivatives of caffeic acid as lipoxygenase inhibitors with antioxidant properties, *Russian Journ. Bioorganic Chemistry*, 21(2): 124–31.

67 Panizzi, L., Pinzauti, M. (1989). The use of propolis in atmospheric disinfection, *Demetra*, (13): 11–13.

68 Grunberger, D., Banerjee, R., Eisinger, K., Oltz, E. M., Efros, L., Caldwell, M., Esteevez, V., Nakanishi, K. (1988). Preferential cytotoxicity on tumour cells by caffeic acid phenethyl ester isolated from propolis, *Experientia (Monthly Journal of Pure and Applied Science)* 44(3): 230–32.

69 Konig, B. (1988). News about propolis: Caffeic acid derivatives responsible for anti-cancer activity and allergy. *Heil Kunst*, 101(1).

70 Scheller, S., Krol, W., Swiacik., Owczarek, S., Gabrys, J., Shani, J. (1989). Anti-tumoral property of ethanolic extract of propolis in mice bearing Ehrlich carcinoma, as compared to bleomycin, *S. Naturforsch(C)*, 44 (11–12): 1063–5.

71 Ross, P. B. (1990). The effects of propolis fractions on cells in tissue cultures. MPhil. thesis, University of Wales College of Cardiff, UK, XII, 193.
72 Matsuno, Tetsuya. (1992). Isolation of the tumoricidal substances from Brazilian propolis, *Honeybee Science*, 13(2): 49–54.
73 Basic, I., Orselic, N., Brbot-Saranovic, A., Tadic, Z., Sulimanovic, D. (1997). XXXVth International Congress Apiculture, 398.
74 Kivalkina, V. P. (1969). Effects of propolis on immunobiological reactivity (abstract), XXIInd International Congress of Apiculture, 463.
75 Dunyavin, A. V. (1971). Adjuvant effect of metal chelate and propolis on immunological reactions of animals in tests of hyper-immunization with paratyphoid antigen, *Uchenye Zapiski Kazanskogo Veterinarnogo Institute*, 109: 158–160.
76 Shevchenko, L. F., Chasovdtseva, O. A., Peschanskii, A. N. (1971). Inhibiting activity of propolis on the influenza virus, *Khimioprofil, Khimioter. Grippa Mater, Vses. Simp*, 1: 56–7.
77 Belozerova, G. A. (1976). Use of propolis to stimulate antibody formation in pigs injected with Aujeszky's disease, *Uchenye Zapiski Kazanskogo Veterinarnogo Institute*, 117: 138–140.
78 Karandoshov, I. G., Kamalov, G., Belozerova, G. A. (1977). Comparison of the immune response of pigs vaccinated with 'BUK-628' live Aujesky's disease vaccine with and without addition of propolis, *Uchenye Zapiski Kazanskogo Veterinarnogo Institute*, 126. 23–7.
79 Esanu, V., Prahoveanu, E., Crisan, I., Cioca, A. (1981). The effects of an aqueous propolis extract, of rutin and of a rutin-quercitin mixture on experimental influenza virus infection in mice (abstract), *Revue Roumaine de Medecine Virologie*, 32(3) 3213–5.
80 Giurgea, R., Poescu, H., Polinicencu. C. (1983). Effects of standardized propolis extract (SPE) on immune reactions, *Clujul Medical*, 56(1) 73–6.
81 Konig, B., Dustmann, J. H. (1985). The caffeoylics as a new family of natural antiviral compounds, *Naturwissenshcaften*, 72 659–62.

82 Konig, B., Dustmann, J. H. (1986). Propolis and viruses: current status of a research project. *Apidologie*, 17(4) 334–6.
83 Neychev, H., Dimoy, V., Vuleva, V., Shirova, L., Slavcheva, E., Geogova, G., Manolova, N., Bankova, V. (1988). Immunomodulatory action of propolis II Effect of water-soluble fraction on influenza infection in mice, *Acta-Microbiol-Bulg*, 23: 58–62.
84 Scheller, S., Gazda, G. (1988). The ability of ethanol extract of propolis to stimulate plaque formation in immunised mouse spleen cells, *Pharmacol, Res.-Commun.*, 20(4): 323–8.
85 Debuaggi, M., Tateo, F., Pagani, L., Lunin, M., Romero, E. (1990). Effects of propolis flavonoids on virus infectivity and replication, *Microbiologica*, 13: 207–13.
86 Amoros, M., Simoes, C. M. O., Girre, L. (1992). Synergistic effect of flavones and flavonols against herpes simplex virus type I in cell culture. Comparison with the antiviral activity of propolis, *J. Nat. Prod.*, 55(12): 1732–40.
87 Serkedjieva, J., Manolova, N. (1992). Anti-influenza virus effect of some propolis constituents and their analogues (esters of substituted cinnamic acids), *J. Nat. Prod.*, 55(3): 294–302.

Chapter 6 Using Propolis to Treat Disease

1 Havsteen, B. cited in Wade, C. (1983). *Propolis: Nature's energizer. Miracle healer from the beehive*, Keats Publishing Inc.
2 McEwan, L. (Allergy specialist) (1994). Propolis (unpublished paper).
3 Christova, V. M. (1986). A propolis enriched wax therapy against inflammatory diseases of the articular muscular system. XXXth International Congress of Apiculture, 429–43.
4 Stoyanka Stoyanova (1997). Wax treatment with propolis of degenerative articular diseases (arthrosis), XXXVth International Congress of Apiculture, 444–5.
5 Mihailescu, N. N. (1975). Physiotherapy in bronchial asthma, cited in *A remarkable hive product: Propolis: Scientific data and suggestions concerning its composition, properties and the possible use in therapeutics*, Apimondia Publishing House.
6 McEwan, L. (Allergy specialist), (1994). (unpublished paper).

7 Serbanescu, T., Palos, E., Boerescu, L., Calcaianu, G. (1975). Propolis alcohol solution (propolis spray) for protecting bed-kept patients from cutaneous infections and bedsores, cited in *A remarkable hive product: Propolis: Scientific data and suggestions concerning its composition, properties and the possible use in therapeutics*, Apimondia Publishing House.
8 Stojko, A., Buczek, E., Siwiec, A., Stojko, J., Koziowsk-Staniczek, J., Hetmanczyk, L. (1999). Use of three per cent Sepropol medication in decubitus ulcer healing, XXXVIth International Congress of Apiculture (Vancouver), 250.
9 Stojko, A. (1978). Biological properties and clinical application of propolis VIII Experimental observation on the influence of ethanol extract of propolis (EEP) on the regeneration of bone tissue. *Arzneimittel-forschung*, 28(1): 35–3.
10 Przybylski, J., Scheller, S. (1985). Early results in the treatment of Legg-Calve-Perthes disease using intra-articular injections of aqueous propolis extract, *Z-Orthop.*, 123(2) 163–7.
11 Rux, V. R. (1975). The treatment with propolis of non-specific endobronchitis, cited in *A remarkable hive product: Propolis: Scientific data and suggestions concerning its composition, properties and the possible use in therapeutics*, Apimondia Publishing House.
12 Scheller, S., Aleksandrowicz, J., Nikodemowicz, E., Czuba, Z. P., Krol, W., Zydowicz, G., Malinowska, B., Keiloch-Szkoda, M. (1989). Trials of immunoregulation in patients with chronic bronchitis, *Immunologica Polska*, 14(3/4) 304–5.
13 Chuhrienko, N. D. (1989). Complex treatment of chronic bronchitis, XXXIInd International Congress of Apiculture, 281.
14 Zabelina, G. F. (1969). Thesis on propolis delivered at K. A. Rachfuss Children's Hospital, USSR, cited in Wade, C. (1983). *Propolis: Nature's energizer. Miracle healer from the beehive*, Keats Publishing Inc.
15 Pakhomov, S. P. 1975. Using propolis for local treatment of burns, cited in *A remarkable hive product: Propolis; Scientific data and suggestions concerning its composition, properties and the possible use in therapeutics*, Apimondia Publishing House.

16 Grochowski, J., Bilinska, M., Stankiewicz, D. (1986). The therapeutic effect of 3 per cent propolis ointment on mice of DBA/2AH breed suffering from skin burns subsequently infected with Pseudomonas aeruginosa, XXXth International Congress of Apiculture, 439–440.
17 Ramos, J., Cuza, L. A., Perez Pineiro, A., Giral Rivera, T. (1997). Honey with propolis mixture (HPM) used to treat burns, XXXVth International Congress of Apiculture, 429–431.
18 Nikolov, St., Todorov, V., Gueorguieva, E., Drianovski, St., Vasilieve, V. (1975). Experiment and clinical results of treatment of acute and chronic colitis with propolis XXVth International Congress of Apiculture.
19 Szmeja, Z. *et al.* (1989) Otorlaryngol Pol., 43: 180.
20 Schmidt, H. *et al.* (1980). *Stomatol. DDR 30:491.* Cited in Bone, K. (1994). Propolis: A natural antibiotic, *Australian J Medical Herbalism* V 6(3):.
21 Varachiu, N., Mateescu, C, Luca, N., Popescu, F., Pirvuh, Gh. (1983). Experimental and clinical studies concentrating the treatment of several periodontal diseases with apitherapeutic products. (Abstract). XXIXth International Congress of Apiculture.
22 Martinez Silveira, G., Gou Gudoy, R., Onatorriente, R., Palmer Ortiz, M. C., Falcon, C. (1986). Preliminary study of the effects of propolis in the treatment of (Spanish) Quoted in Compact Cambridge: MEDLINE 1986, (rev. 1990).
23 Neumann, D. (1986). Clinical study of a test of the plaque and gingivitis-inhibiting effects of propolis, *Stomatol-DDR*, 36(12): 677–81.
24 Ibricevic, H., Kostic, A., Krnjic, J. (1987). A study of blood flow in dental pulp of dogs under the influence of propolis and calxyl employing the hydrogen wash-out method, *Acta Stomatologica Croatia*, 21(1): 3–8.
25 Tomaskova, L., Hornova, J., Sindelka, Z., Ondrujova, E., Fassmann, A. (1988). Healing of injured tooth pulp in calf teeth after direct capping with propolis (6 weeks), *Acta Facultatis Med. Univ. Brunensis*, 98: 123–34.
26 Gafar. M., Dumitriu, H., Dumitriu, S., Guti, L. (1989). Apiphytotherapeutic original preparations in the treatment of chronic

marginal parodentopathies. A clinical and microbiological study, *Stomatologie*, 36(2) 91–7.

27 Kosenko, S. V., Kosovich, T. I. (1990). *Stomatologila* 69:27. Cited in Bone, K. (1994) Propolis: A natural antibiotic. *Australian J Medical Herbalism*, 6(3).

28 Ionita, R. (1990). Experimentation of apiarian preparations for the direct and indirect capping of the dental pulp, *Stomotologie*, 37(1): 19–30.

29 Ikeno, K., Ikeno, T., Miyazawa, C. (1991). Effects of propolis on dental caries in rats, *Caries Res.*, 25(5): 347–351.

30 Wander, P. (1995). Taking the sting out of dentistry, *Dental Practice*, 1995 April.

31 Varley P. (1996). Homoepathy in dentistry. A presentation of ten cases for the Dental MFHon Examination.

32 Hai Liu, Fu, Ding Xu, Zheng. (1997). Propolis curing diabetes clinical effect observation. XXXVth International Congress of Apiculture, 417.

33 Gao Hai-lin, Meng Pei-de, Liu Fu-hai, Xu Zheng-ding (1997). 'Fengzhen' Curing diabetes effect and mechanism discussion. XXXVth International Congress of Apiculture, 405.

34 Baidan, N., Oita, N., Palos, E. (1978). Using propolis in ophthalmology, cited in *A remarkable hive product: Propolis: Scientific data and suggestions concerning its composition, properties and the possible use in therapeutics*, Apimondia Publishing House.

35 Popescu, M. P., Popescu, A. (1997). Treatment of ocular cataract by means of the hive products, applied as molecular mycelia. Results of 21 years' of practice. XXXVth International Congress of Apiculture, 428.

36 Iojris, N. P. (1954). *Healing Properties of Honey and Bee Pollen*, USSR Federal Publishing House for Medicine.

37 Shevchenko, L. F. *et al.* (1971). *Khimioprofil, Kimioter Grippa.* 1:56 Cited in Bone, K. Propolis: A natural antibiotic, *Australian J Medical Herbalism*, 6(3).

38 Esanu, V., Prahoveanu, E., Crisan, I., Cioca, A. (1981). The effects of an aqueous propolis extract, of rutin and of a rutin-quercetin mixture on experimental influenza virus infection in mice, *Revue Roumaine de Medecine. Virologie*, 32(3): 213–5.

39 Neychev, H., Dimoy, V., Vuleva, V., Shriova, L., Slavcheva, E., Gegova, G., Manolova, N., Bankova, V. (1988). Immunomodulatory action of propolis. II Effect of water-soluble fraction on influenza infection in mice, *Acta-Microbiol-Bulg*., 23: 58–62.

40 Osmanagic, Izet. (1976). Report of the preventive properties of propolis against influenza, Sarajevo.

41 Ceplak, A., Matjasic, M. (1978). Viricidal effects of Apikompleks during an influenza epidemic, *Slovenski Cebela*, 80(11): 399–400.

42 Fang Chu, (1979). Workers Hospital of Lienyunkan, Kiangsu Province People's Republic of China. Cited in *American Chiropractor*, 2(2).

43 Kovalik, P. V. (1979). The use of propolis in the treatment of patients with chronic fungal sinusitis, *Vestnik Otorinolaringologii*, (6) 60–2.

44 Makarov, F. D. (1972). Propolis Therapy—The Healing Art. USSR No. 4, 190.

45 Omarov, S. M., Omarova, Z. M. (1997). The use of propolis when treating lingering forms of intestinal infections in early childhood. XXXVth. International Congress of Apiculture, 426.

46 Hamanaka, H., Harada, M. (1990). Propolis food compositions containing polyols and polyol fatty acid esters and their manufacture. Japanese Patent (JP 02 245 159 Nippon Propoarisu. K. K. Japan).

47 Chauvin, R. (1980). Use of propolis in treatment of hay fever. Pharmacological assays, *Apiacta*, 15(3) 101–3.

48 Perhakov, I. T. (1973). The Treatment of hypohearing with propolis, *Pcelovodstvo*, 93(3): 38–90.

49 Popnikolov, P., Pochinkova, P., Donchev, St. (1975). The treatment of mesotympanitis with propolis. Cited in *A remarkable hive product: Propolis: Scientific data and suggestions concerning its composition, properties and the possible use in therapeutics*, Apimondia Publishing House.

50 Kachny, G. G. (1975). Treatment with propolis of acute inflammations of the inner ear. Cited in: *A remarkable hive product: Propolis: Scientific data and suggestions concerning its composition, properties and the possible use in the therapeutics*, Apimondia Publishing House.

51 Feiks, Franz Klemens (1978). Topical application of propolis tincture in the treatment of herpes zoster. Third International Symposium on Apitherapy, Portoroz, Yugoslavia, 109–10.
52 Giurcaneanu, F., Crisan, I., Esanu, V., Cioca, V., Cajal, N. (1988). Treatment of cutaneous herpes and herpes zoster with Nivcreisol-D, *Virologie*, 39(1): 1–24.
53 Sven Arne Ring (1995). Antiviral complex of flavonoids from propolis in the treatment of herpes infections, *Journal of Alternative and Complementary Medicine*, (1) 9.
54 Fang Chu. (1979) Workers Hospital of Lienyunkan, Kiangsu Province People's Republic of China. Cited in *American Chiropractor*, 2(2).
55 Olczyk, D., Sojko, R., Stojko, A. (1999). Influence of Sepol—the standardized honey-propolis-pollen extract on cholesterol levels in research conditions. XXXVIth International Congress of Apiculture, 251.
56 Havsteen B. (1988). Personal interview quoted in Wade, C. (1983). *Propolis: Nature's energizer. Miracle healer from the beehive*, Keats Publishing Inc.
57 McEwan, L. (Allergy specialist) (1994). (unpublished paper).
58 Propolis—ME Survey. Conducted by ME Association 1997. Results sent privately to author.
59 Report from Florence Mhonie, Executive Director of ACOBOS, part of the Kenyan National Aids Control Programme. (1996) Produced privately for the author.
60 Kolev, J., Dimtcheva, V. (1997). Beeswax with propolis treatment on patients having low back pain. XXXVth International Congress of Apiculture, 413.
61 Stoyanka, Stoynova. (1999). Beeswax with propolis treatment on patients having low back pain. (abstract) XXXVIth International Congress of Apiculture, 252.
62 Miyares, C., Holands, I., Castaneda, C., Gonzalez, T., Fragoso, T., Curras, R., Soria, C. (1988). Clinical trials with a preparation based on propolis 'Propolisina' in human giardiasis, *Acta Gastroenterol. Latinoam*, 18(3): 195–201.
63 Kravchuk, I. A. (1971). Results of use of a propolis extract for chronic subatrophic and atrophic pharyngitis, *Zh. Ushn-Nos–Bolezn*, 31(1): 73–78.

64 Doroshenko, P. N. (1975). Propolis and chronic pharyngitis. *Propolis: Scientific data and suggestions concerning its composition, properties and the possible use in therapeutics*, Apimondia Publishing House.

65 Popovici, C., Saranga, M. (1975). Treatment with propolis and other hive products of some otorhinolaryngological affections. *Propolis: Scientific data and suggestions concerning its composition, properties and the possible use in therapeutics*, Apimondia Publishing House.

66 Matel, I., Straka, J., Cizmarik, J. (1975). Effects of propolis in otorhinolaryngology. *Propolis: Scientific data and suggestions concerning its composition, properties and the possible use in therapeutics*, Apimondia Publishing House.

67 Mladenov, S., Mladenova, D. S. (1997). Prostate adenoma apitherapy. XXXVth International Congress of Apiculture, 425.

68 Saraf, A. L., Souvorov, A., Concharuk, A. (1999). New complex bee medicine Prostapin in the treatment of urologic and gynaecologic diseases. (abstract) XXXVIth International Congress of Apiculture, 247.

69 Osmanagic, I., Beljenki, D., Mavric, N. (1979). Treatment with propolis of irradiation diseases. Cited in *American Chiropractor*, 2(2).

70 Zabelina, G. F. (1969). Thesis on propolis delivered at K. A. Rachfuss Children's Hospital, USSR. Cited in Wade, C. (1983). *Propolis: Nature's energizer. Miracle healer from the beehive*, Keats Publishing Inc.

71 Danilov, L. N. (1975). Treatment of some skin diseases with propolis. *Propolis: Scientific data and suggestions concerning its composition, properties and the possible use in therapeutics*, Apimondia Publishing House.

72 Vinogradova, T. V., Zajceva, (1979), G. P. Cited in *American Chiropractor*, 2(2).

73 Lauda E. Cited in Wade, C. (1983). *Propolis: Nature's energizer. Miracle healer from the beehive*, Keats Publishing Inc.

74 McEwan, L. (Allergy specialist) (1994). Propolis (unpublished paper).

75 Krylov, V., Oshevensky, L., Kurnikov, G., Klemenova, I. (1999). Cream based on wax with propolis and royal jelly in the treatment of dermatological diseases. (abstract) XXXVIth International Congress of Apiculture, 249.
76 Krivoruchko, V. P., Degtyarenko, V. I., Zaitseva, T. I., Ganchenko, M. G. (1975). Anti-viral effects of propolis, *Virusy I Virusnye Zaboleyaniya*, 3: 61–4.
77 Karimova, Z. H., Rodionova, E. I. (1975). Propolis in complex treatment of pulmonary tuberculosis. *Propolis: Scientific data and suggestions concerning its composition, properties and the possible use in therapeutics*, Apimondia Publishing House.
78 Kurilin, I A., Shamrai, T. E. (1972). Treatment with propolis of complicated trephination cavities after surgical operations and tympanoplasty, *Vestnik Otorinolarinoologii*, 34(2) 57–9.
79 Feiks, F. K. (1978). Propolis extracts in the treatment of ulcer affections, Third International Symposium on Apitherapy, Portoroz, Yugoslavia, 319–22 (German) pp. 322–23 (English) (abstract).
80 Korsun, V. F. (1983) Use of propolis in the treatment of trophic ulcers, *Vestn.-Dermatol,-Venerol*, (11): 46–8.
81 Gorbatenko, A. G. (1971). Treatment of ulcer patients with a 30% alcohol solution of propolis, *Vrach.-Delo*, (3): 22–4.
82 Vasilca, A., Milcu, E. (1975). Local treatment of chronic ulcers with extract of propolis. *Propolis: Scientific data and suggestions concerning its composition, properties and the possible use in therapeutics*, Apimondia Publishing House.
83 McEwan, L. (Allergy specialist) (1994). Propolis (unpublished paper).
84 Dept Obstetrics Kiev Hospital. Cited in Wade. C. (1983). *Propolis: Nature's energizer. Miracle healer from the beehive.* Keats Publishing Inc.
85 Brusilovskij, I. A., Vinogradova, T. V., Zajceva, G. P. Cited Wade. C. (1983) *Propolis: Nature's energizer. Miracle healer from the beehive.* Keats Publishing Inc.
86 Zwadadzki, J., Suchy, H., Scheller, S. (1973). Use of propolis for treatment of vaginitis and cervicitis (author's translation), *Przegl-Lek.* 30(7): 629–33. Cited in *Propolis*, Apimondia Publishing House, *Bucharest*, 1975. 175–7.

87 Suchy, H., Scheller, S. (1975). Results of propolis in gynaecology. *Propolis*, Apimondia Publishing House, *Bucharest*, 1975, 175–7.
88 Roman, S., Mateescu, C., Palos, E. (1989). Treatment of some gynaecological diseases with apitherapeutics. International Congress of Apiculture.
89 Cheakova, Z. (1997). Observations on the use of propolis, under the form of ion-therapy and ultrasound therapy in patients suffering from cervical arthrosis. XXXVth International Congress of Apiculture, 400.
90 Panova, Z., Vassilev, V. (1997). Use of propolis for treating some gynaecological diseases. XXXVth International Congress of Apiculture, 428.
91 Scheller, S. *et al. Przeglad Lekasrski* 37:739. Cited in Bone, K. (1994) Propolis: A natural anitbiotic, *Aust. J. Med. Herbalism* 6 (3).
92 Damyanliev, R., Hekimov, K., Savova, E., Agopian, R. (1982). The treatment of suppurative surgical wounds with propolis, *Folia-Med. (Plovdiv)*, 24(2): 24–27.
93 Tsarev, N. I. *et al. Veestn. Khir*, 134: 119. Cited in Bone, K. (1994) Propolis: A natural antibiotic, *Aust. J. Med. Herbalism* 6 (3).
94 Przbylski, J., Scheller, S. (1985). Early results in the treatment of Legg—Calve—Perthe disease using intra-articular injections of aqueous propolis extract, *Z-Orthop*. 123(2): 163–7.

Chapter 7 Propolis Products and their Use

1 McEwan, L. (Allergy specialist) (1994). Propolis (unpublished paper).
2 Murat, F. (1982). *Propolis—The Eternal Natural Healer*, privately published.
3 Propolis—ME. Conducted by UK ME Association (1994) private communication to the author.
4 Murat, F. (1982). *Propolis—The Eternal Natural Healer*, privately published.
5 *ibid.*
6 *ibid.*

7 *ibid.*
8 Kivalkina, V. P., Gorshunova, V. I. (1973). The possibility to use propolis combined with antbiotics (abstract), *Antibiotika* (Moscow), 18(3): 261–3.
9 Murat, F. (1982). *Propolis—The Eternal Natural Healer*, privately published.
10 *ibid.*
11 Jolly, V. B. (1977). Propolis violin varnish. *Strad.*, 88(1052): 713, 715, 717, 719.
12 Murat, F. (1982). *Propolis—The Eternal Natural Healer*, privately published.
13 Ogren. American Patent.
14 Murat, F. (1982). *Propolis—The Eternal Natural Healer*, privately published.

Chapter 8 Propolis and Animals

1 Yang, Ruiya *et al.* (1989). The effects and use of propolis on veterinary medicine. XXXIIIrd International Congress of Apiculture.
2 (USSR Ministry of Agriculture) (1978). Veterinary applications of propolis, *Veterinariya Moscow, USSR* 12:106–108.
3 Mirolyubov, M. G., Barskov, A. A. (1980). Propolis and mastitis, *Veterinariya Moscow, USSR* 2: 45–6.
4 Meresta, L., Meresta, T., (1985). At attempt to use propolis extract in the treatment of mastitis of cows, *Medycyna Weterynaryja*, 45(7): 392–5.
5 Meresta, T., Burdzinski, J., Chmurzynski, P. (1989). Treatment of mastitis in cows using an extract of propolis, *Medycyna Weterynaryja*, 45(7): 392–5.
6 Khramov, A. V. (1984) Effects of propolis on the uterine contractions of cows, *Veterinariya, Moscow USSR*, 2: 52–53.
7 Dunyavin, A. V. (1971). Adjuvant effect of metal chelate and propolis on immunological reactions of animals in tests of hyperimmunization with paratyphoid antigen, *Uchenye Zapiski Kazanskogo Veterinarnogo Institute*, 109: 158–160.
8 Teterev, T. I. (1972). Effect of propolis on the synthesis of specific agglutinins, *Veterinariya Moscow, USSR* 48(3): 41–2.

9 Tomaskova, L., Hornova, J., Sindelka, Z., Ondrujova, E., Fassman, A. (1988). Healing of injured tooth pulp in calf teeth after direct capping with propolis (6 weeks), *Acta Facultatis Med. Univ. Brunensis*, 98: 123–134.

10 Lori, G. A. (1990). Fungicidal effect of propolis in bovine dermatomycosis, *Industria Apicola* 1(1):38–43.

11 Budicza, A., Molnar, P. (1987). Propolis in the rearing of calves, *Mezoqazdasag*, 42(17): 14.

12 Belozerova, G. A. (1976). Inhibitory effect of propolis on Aujeszky's disease virus *in vitro*, *Uchenye Zapiski Kazanskogo Verinarnogo Institute*, 122: 58–62.

13 Myung-Sang Kwon, Ji-Min Kim, Young-Jae Kim, Jung Yoon Kim, Zhong-Zhe Han, Hwan Lim. (1999). Use of propolis in neonatal diarrhoea in calves, XXXVIth International Congress of Apiculture, 248.

14 Belozerova, G. A. (1976). Use of propolis to stimulate antibody formation in pigs vaccinated against Aujeszky's disease, *Uchenye Zapiski Kazanskogo Verinarnogo Institute*, 117: 138–40.

15 Karanddashov, I. G., Kamalov, G. Kh., Belozerova, G. A. (1977). Comparison of the immune response of pigs vaccinated with 'BUK-628' live Aujeszky's disease vaccine, with or without the addition of propolis.

16 Buhatel, T., Vesa, S., Sabau, A. L., Dimitriu, A., Modovan, I. (1983). Contribution to the knowledge of the stimulative effect of propolis on piglets and pullets.

17 Bonomi, A., Marletto, F., Bianchi, M. (1976). Use of propolis in the food of laying hens, *Rivista di Avicoltura*, 45(4): 43–55.

18 Sutta, J., Hanko, J., Janda, J., Tkac, J. (1974). Experimental and clinical experience in the treatment of wounds in domestic animals by local application of an alcohol solution of propolis, *Folia Veterinaria*, 18(1/2): 143–7.

19 Munoz Larriera, B. (1989). Prevention of legs infections in bovines using propolis. *Apiacta*, 24(3) 80–81.

20 Tsakov, Ts. (1975). Study on the local anaesthetic characteristics of propolis and their effect in operations on sheep and dogs. *Propolis*, Apimondia Publishing House, 67.

21 Hollands, I., Miyares, C., Sigarroa, A., Perez, A. (1984).

Efficacy of propolis against infection by intestinal *Eimeria* in rabbits, *Rivista Cubana de Ciencias Veterinarias*, 15(2): 157–163.
22 Hollands, I., Miyares, C., Siogarroa, A. (1988). Comparative analysis of the action of propolis, sulphaqunioxaline and suplhamethazine in rabbits with coccidiosis, *Rivista Cubana de Ciencias Veterinarias*, 19(2): 99–104.
23 Ikeno, K., Ikeno, T., Miyazawa, C. (1991). Effects of propolis on dental caries in rats, *Caries Res.*, 25(5): 347–51.

Chapter 9 Propolis—The Impact of Commercial Exploitation

1 *Here's Health Magazine*, March 1993.
2 The *Sun*, March 1994.
3 Ochi, T. (1981). A new method for collecting propolis, *Honeybee Science*, 2(1): 16.
4 Andrich, G., Fiorentini, R., Consglieri, A. (1987). Characteristics of some examples of propolis from the Ligurian coast, *Citta delle Api*, 28: 30–31.
5 Marletto, F. (1983). Characteristics of propolis in terms of its floral origin and its use by honeybees, *Apiacta*, 19(3): 71–4.
6 Krell, R. (1996). Value added products from Beekeeping. *FAO Agricultural Services Bulletin*, 124.
7 *ibid.*
8 *ibid.*
9 Nikolov, *et al.* (1987). Romanian Patent.
10 EPID, Verona, Italy.
11 Russian Quality Standards for Propolis (1977). cited in Krell, R. Value added products from beekeeping. *FAO Agricultural Services Bulletin*, 124.
12 See HFMA (Health Food Manufacturers Association) Propolis Standard (1995).

Chapter 10 Making Your Own Medicines

1 Krell, R. (1996). Value added products from Beekeeping. *FAO Agricultural Services Bulletin*, 124.

2 *ibid.*

3 Kaal, J. (1991). *Natural Medicine from Honey Bees*, Kaal Printing House.

4 Senghali

5 Kaal, J. (1991). *Natural Medicine from Honey Bees*, Kaal Printing House.

6 *ibid.*

7 *ibid.*

8 Murat, F. (1982). *Propolis—The Eternal Natural Healer*, privately published.

9 Sonowski, cited in Krell, R. (1996). Value added products from Beekeeping. *FAO Agricultural Services Bulletin*, 124.

10 Krochmal, cited in Krell, R. (1996). Value added products from Beekeeping. *FAO Agricultural Services Bulletin*, 124.

11 Murat, F. (1982). *Propolis—The Eternal Natural Healer*, privately published.

12 Sonowski, cited in Krell, R. (1996). Value added products from Beekeeping. *FAO Agricultural Services bulletin*, 124.

13 Murat, F. (1982). *Propolis—The Eternal Natural Healer*, privately published.

14 *ibid.*

15 Lejeune, quoted in Krell, R. (1996). Value added products from Beekeeping. *FAO Agricultural Services Bulletin*, 124.

APPENDIX 1

Health Food Manufacturers Propolis Specification

HARVESTED RAW PROPOLIS

Description

Propolis is a resinous substance of botanical origin collected and modified by bees.

Appearance

Resinous/waxy substance.

Colour

Variable according to origin, generally through shades from light to dark green-brown or red-brown/black.

Organoleptic

Characteristic aromatic aroma; variable according to origin. Generally mildly numbing effect when placed on the tongue.

Identifiers

	Test Method
The following flavonoids must be detectable using High Performance Liquid Chromatography (HPLC):	A1
Chrysin	
Pinocembrin	
Galangin	

Purity

		Test Method
Wax content	50% w/w maximum	A2(a)
Total Ash	5% w/w maximum	A3

Chemical Composition and Identification

Flavonoid content:		A1
Chrysin	1% w/w minimum	
Pinocembrin	1% w/w/ minimum	
Galangin	1% w/w minimum	

Harvested Raw Propolis sold direct to the ultimate consumer

Must fulfil all the above criteria, plus

Lead content	1 mg/kg maximum	A5(a)
Arsenic content	1 mg/kg maximum	A5(b)

PURIFIED RAW PROPOLIS

Description

Purified raw propolis is the total alcohol and/or water extracted matter obtained from raw propolis meeting the relevant standard, with addition of no further ingredients.

Colour

Light/dark brown to black.

Appearance

A resinous substance.

Organoleptic

Characteristic aromatic odour. Generally mildly numbing effect when placed on the tongue.

Identifiers

	Test Method
The following flavonoids must be detectable	A1

using High Performance Liquid Chromatography (HPLC):
Chrysin
Pinocembrin
Galangin

Purity

		Test Method
Wax content	5% w/w maximum	A2(b)
Total Ash	2% w/w maximum	A3
Loss on drying	5% w/w maximum	A4
Lead content	1 mg/kg maximum	A5(a)
Arsenic content	1 mg/kg maximum	A5(b)

Chemical Composition and Identification

Flavonoid content:		A1
Chrysin	2% w/w minimum	
Pinocembrin	2% w/w/ minimum	
Galangin	2% w/w minimum	

APPENDIX 2

Test Method A1

METHOD FOR FLAVONOID ANALYSIS IN PROPOLIS BY HPLC

Introduction

This method is intended for the quantitative analysis of chrysin, galangin and pinocembrin in raw and purified propolis by tincturing in ethanol and subsequent HPLC. The data can be used to set specifications or for quality control purposes.

Sample Preparation

Finely shave or cut the sample if not in existing powdered form. Prepare a 10% tincture by accurately weighing five grams solid into a 50 ml volumetric flask and topping up near to the mark with ethanol (95%). Shake well and ultrasonicate the solution for one hour, with periodic shaking. Top up to the mark, mix well and leave to stand at room temperature overnight (lesser amounts than five grams may be taken, but in view of the poor homogeneity of propolis resin 5 g is recommended. If this cannot be done, a *minimum* of 1 g should be taken).

Next day, shake again and allow gross material to settle. Dilute 400 μl of this solution to 10 ml in a volumetric flask with ethanol and filter through a 0.45 μ filter (e.g. Gelgam LC13). If using an autopipette to dispense the volume, beware the lower viscosity of ethanol compared to water and the consequent propensity for drips. Take care also not to block the pipette tip with solid material. Discard the initial one ml filtrate and introduce the remainder into a capped vial for HPLC.

Standards

The flavonoids are purchased from Extrasynthese (Lyon, France) and individual stock standard solutions are made up in ethanol at 100 ppm as follows:

Quercetin, chrysin	50 mg to 50 ml
Galangin, pinocembrin (more costly)	10 mg to 10 ml

These are then diluted further in ethanol (one ml to 20) to give a mixed working standard containing approximately 50 ppm of each component. Stock standards and mixed standards may be kept tightly closed in the deep freeze—it is convenient to keep the working standard pre-prepared in individual HPLC vials for immediate use.

HPLC Conditions

The following conditions are those used in the RSSL laboratory. Other equipment and columns may be used with appropriate modifications to obtain satisfactory resolution of the three key analytes chrysin, galangin and pinocembrin.

Equipment: Hewlett-Packard HP 1090 with diode array detection
Column: Phenomenex Columbus C18 150 mm × 4.6 mm
Temperature: 45°C
Flow rate: 1 ml/min
Injection: 10 µl
Solvent A: 5% formic acid in water
Solvent B: Methanol
Gradient:

Time	%A	%B
0	65	35
45	20	80
50	5	95
55	65	35
65	65	35

Detection wavelengths:
268 nm—chrysin and galangin
280 nm—pinocembrin
350 nm—quercetin

Peaks are checked for identity by retention time and diode-array spectral match. Quantification for each peak is performed at the appropriate wavelength with reference to the appropriate external standard which is run at the beginning and end of a batch. On the equipment shown, linearity of standard response was demonstrated between 20–150 ppm (as injected) for each of the three major analytes.

To express the flavonoids as parts per million (mg/kg) in the original propolis, a multiplication factor of approximately 250 should be used (calculated accurately from the weight of propolis taken). To express the flavonoids in percent w/w, as in this study, the multiplication factor is *ca* 2.5×10^{-2}.

A note on column performance

Over a period of time, resin from the propolis appears to deposit on the HPLC column and degrades resolution and performance. For this reason, the use of an appropriate guard column is recommended. It is also advisable to flush the column with acetonitrile after use, followed by occasional washing with dichloromethane to remove accumulated wax and resin. The column should then be washed again with acetonitrile prior to storage.